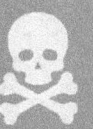

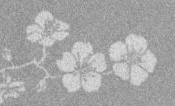

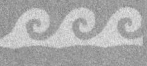

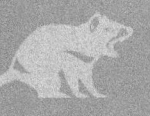

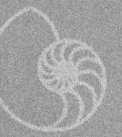

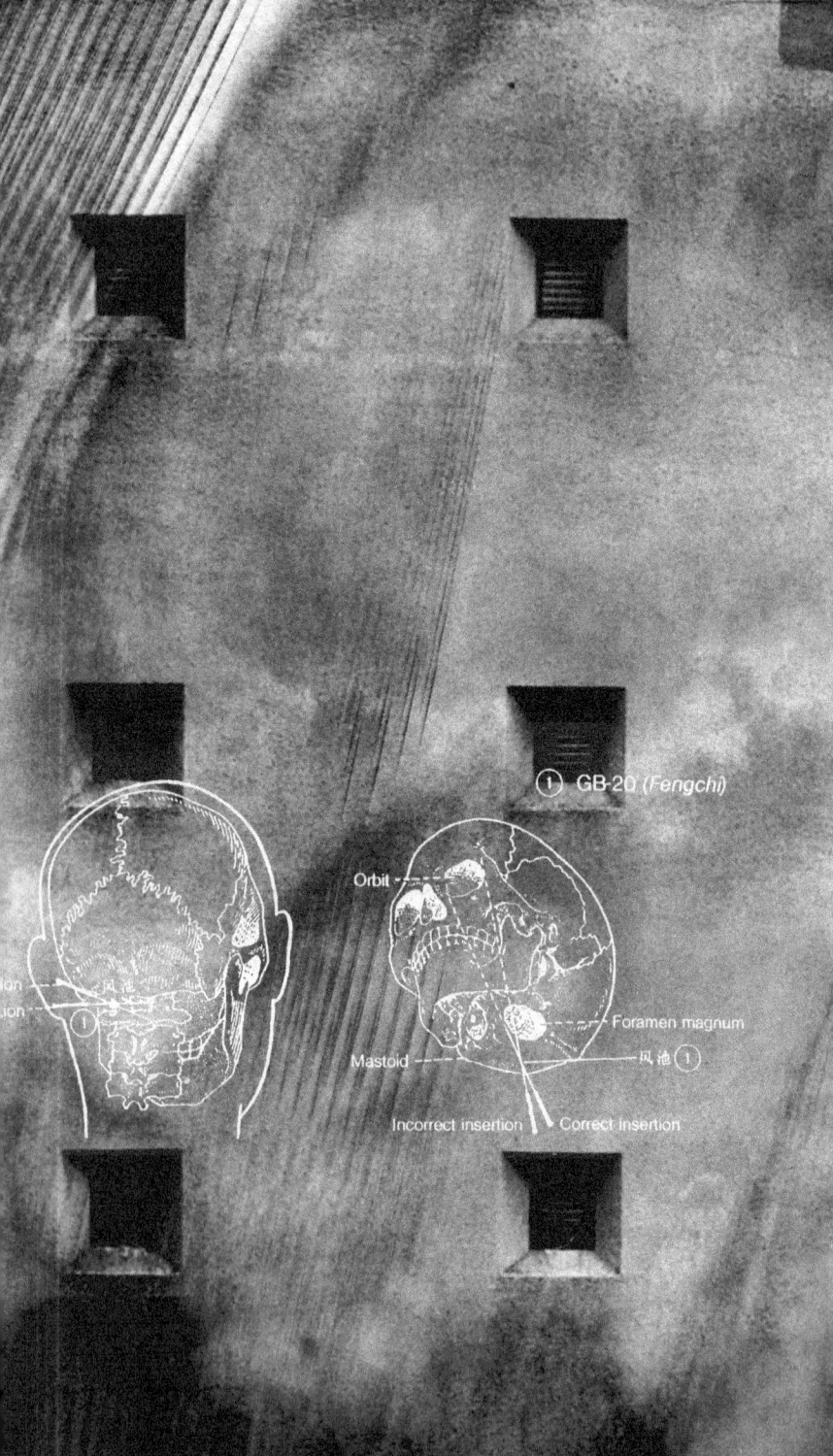

The Evolve Restoration Series
by Beth Alderman, MD, MPH

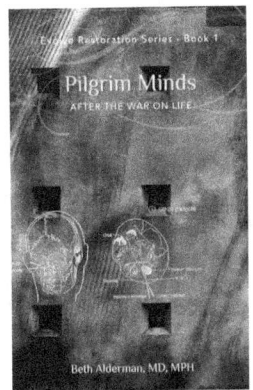

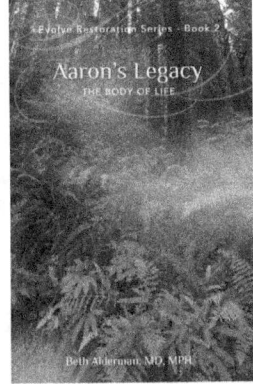

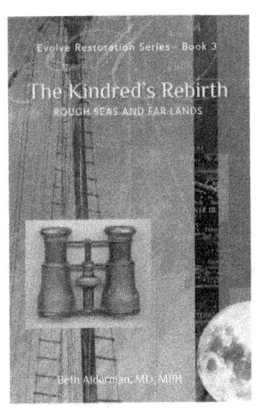

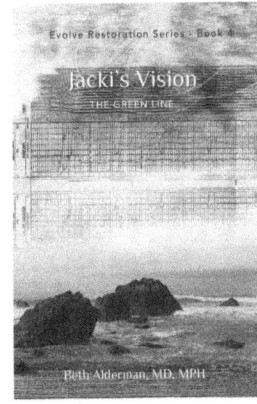

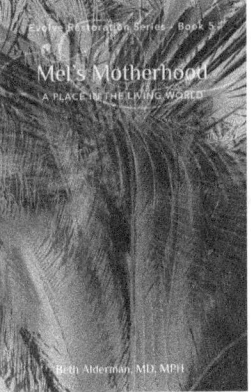

Pilgrim Minds

AFTER THE WAR ON LIFE

Book One of the
Evolve Restoration Series

Beth Alderman

FUTURE MEDICINE LLC · ASHLAND, OREGON

Pilgrim Minds: After the War on Life
by Beth Alderman, MD, MPH
© 2019 Beth Alderman
www.LivingFutureBooks.com
For related online courses visit
www.LivingFutureCourses.com

Editor: Julie Clayton
Cover Art: BruceBayard.com
Book Design: BookSavvyStudio.com

Library of Congress Control Number: 2019903854
ISBN: 978-1-7321110-5-9
First Edition
Printed in the United States of America

Contents

To Cynthia, Ted, and Jamal

How sour sweet music is when time is broke and no proportion kept. So it is in the music of men's lives … I wasted time, and now doth time waste me.

— SHAKESPEARE, King Richard II

There are many events in the womb of time which will be delivered.

—SHAKESPEARE, Othello

Columbus, the very same man whose arrival in the Caribbean touched off a landslide of deforestation from which Ayiti has never recovered … noted that 'now that the many woods and trees that covered [the Azores] have been felled, there are not produced so many clouds and rains as before.' These observations were, however, insufficient to protect Ayiti's magnificent hardwoods, which were pillaged by the shipload."

—APRICOT IRVING

1

Pilgrims

As Aaron lathers his brush on the bar of shaving soap and thinks back over the past few days of sitting at his mother's bedside in their clinic hospice, he feels overcome. He leans on the old sink, soap brush dangling between his thumb and forefinger. He has been too tired to think, and too distressed not to ruminate on these last days and minutes of the life of his best friend, closest companion, and most trusted advisor.

Aaron moves to distract himself by shaving his cowlicky stubble. He whets his blade on the strop, runs hot water on a cloth, and steams his face. When he looks in the mirror, he does not recognize himself. The wide eyes and deep frown of grief bring his father's ingrained resentment to life, as does the prominent chin that a willful high school sweetheart called a sign of stubbornness. The rest of his face is his mother's: the full head of sandy hair graying at the temples, the high forehead, broad cheekbones, full lips, and ski nose. He is his parents now. This thought is paradoxically calming; it brings him back to himself. He sighs in relief. He needs this.

Last night after napping in his bed, he returned to the hospice and found his mother clasping the hand of an old stranger who sat on her bed as if he belonged at her side. As Aaron watched, the stranger bent down to give his mother a long kiss on the lips, after which her face glowed as if she were a young girl who had just met her first love. Her eyes opened and she spoke with the man at length. Feeling as if he were looking at two strangers, Aaron retreated to the staff room and sat on the high stool beyond the kitchenette to think.

She must have met someone after Dad died, someone she saw when she traveled.

There, in the gentle light of the high windows beneath the eaves, surrounded by the fronds and flowers of the living wall, he listened to the sad or stoic murmurs coming from the hospice and felt the walls stifle him. Eyes on the floor, he stood and sped up the central hall of the clinic, between examining rooms and hothouses, past doors to care suites and residences, and out the front door into the cold spring morning.

He turned right, rounded the corner, and paused at a bench, where his wild eyes caught those of a passing neighbor who nodded respectfully and moved on. Aaron was in no fit state to speak with any of the long-time friends and neighbors who shared his grief. He turned to the well-mulched rose bushes behind which his father was interred, and reached up to touch the granite tile on the outwide wall that reads "Dr. Daniel Aboulafia, 1954-2033, Iowa City, Iowa." His father kept to the old place name so that he would, he had explained sardonically, know where he was.

His mother's plaque, already in place around the corner, beside the hospice door in the back, reads "Dr. Melissa Sundquist Aboulafia, 1955-2050, Residential Habitat Restoration Clinic, Amana group, Missouria bioregion." Aaron strode to it, stared at it, sighed, and sat beside it on a backless bench, elbows on his knees, face to the ground, breathing out evanescent puffs of steam.

"Aaron?" asked a gentle voice, breaking his reverie.

Aaron looked up to find the stranger standing in front of the bench, hand extended. Taking it, Aaron shook it reluctantly. He tried to read the stranger, but saw only old age: fallen features, bottle-lensed glasses dangling on a string, sound-editing ear inserts, sunken chest and sagging belly girdled with a belted coat. The man leaned on a hand-carved cane with a four-point tip. He continued in a high voice strained by pent emotion.

"I'm John. I was there at the Saltspring Island Research Station in 2010, and met you and your brother. You look the same to me, just like your mother did at your age."

Meeting the man's gaze, Aaron found it intensely loving and therefore unnerving in a stranger.

"I'm sorry, I don't remember."

"I started a clinic similar to yours in New York, in Ithaca."

Aaron studied John's face while asking in as neutral a tone as he could, "Why don't I know you? I set up all the conference calls."

At that, John looked away, his eyes reddening. "We lost touch, and later caught up at meetings." He began to choke back tears. "I'm sorry. It's too much for both of us, I can see. Let's talk more later. I'll come by the comm tower." He turned abruptly and headed across the frozen lawn toward the guesthouse, his gait strong but his balance unsteady, saying *sotto voce*, "He should have been my son."

Now, as Aaron is shaving his Adam's apple, he nicks it, abruptly remembering when he saw John forty years earlier, when the older man was tall and lithe. Aaron and his brother Eric were flanking their father Dan, facing John and his three children—a girl and two boys in their teens, if Aaron remembers rightly. John had dark hair like Dan's, but straight and fine instead of curly. He had green eyes; a long face; a more prominent mouth, now obscured by his old man nose; and a cleft chin. John's expression had been somber and Dan's had been characteristically angry;

Aaron and Eric had instinctively fallen in line and faced John as an intruder. Aaron didn't understand it then, but now he recognizes that his father must have been jealous. John must have been an old boyfriend from the medical school where his parents met.

He must have missed their communications. Lately, he has been absorbed by life in the Amanas, which has sustained its transparent peaceful state as if the madness of late modernity had never taken place, as if they had only been waiting for technology to catch up with their ability to share life and love through prayer.

Aaron throws on his hat and jacket, steps into his boots, and exits the communications tower where he has lived out most of his life. As he walks, he realizes that the breeze is chafing his numb ears. Belatedly, he pulls up the collar of his pigskin jacket and folds down the earflaps of his fur-lined cap before making his way back to the hospice door. He passes thick-knuckled farmers, farmwives, and sturdy children walking toward the dining place from their German pietist church. It must be Sunday.

When his family moved here from Denver, he had made nothing of what he saw; now its culture and roots have become his. The history of those who farm here extends back to the Ebenezer colony of the early 1800's and the radical reformation before that. The furrowed fields before him hearken back to the dawn of human cultivation. His parents' lineages are as old, of course, and he can trace them back for millennia. Aaron's father's lineage goes back through Sephardic roots to the time of Nehemiah; his mother's back through the time of Swedenborg to the burial mounds of the Vikings and their ancestors.

Yet all of Aaron's personal history has matured here. He has lived out his solitary life enclosed by this island of humanity that gave his family refuge and made them welcome. For the past forty years, this community and its roots and his family's have comprised the whole of his world. He can barely imagine what it would be like to leave.

He returns to his mother's bedside now and removes his outer garb again. She is lying flat, her white hair loose on the pillow, her crusted lips nearly colorless. He waits for his hands to warm and then takes hers gently in his. Her archaic smile remains placid, her hands still. Sitting down in the soft recliner beside the bed, he continues his vigil, watching her bony chest rise and fall with her breath.

Aaron's head nods. He falls into a doze during which he jerks his head up from time to time. He notices John's coat come and go from the bench at the foot of the bed. Later, he comes to and finds his mother staring at him. She opens her hand to him; he takes it. He moves to sit beside her on the bed.

"I want to give you my blessing now, and to leave you with my last wish."

He clasps her hand tightly, swallows his tears, and kneels on the floor by her pillow. She puts her hand on his head and mutters gratitudes, praises, hopes, and love in Aramaic and in English. When she finishes and puts her hand on his cheek, he says formally, "Thank you, Mother, for life and love."

"And you, my dear son," she says with a beatific smile.

"And your wish?" he asks. He is barely able to contain his emotion now despite all the spiritual practice that she taught him. Some time elapses before he catches her words and struggles to wrap his sodden mind around them. He looks into her intense gaze, absorbs her urgent desperation, and comprehends that her last wish is a doozy. She wants him, the only communicator in the Amana Colonies, who has only a tiny store of credits to his name, to travel two thousand miles to see her friend Sarah and accept his legacy—whatever that is. When he promises to do it, and then asks what it is, she lays back, relieved and spent, and slides into oblivion.

Aaron is non-plussed; he wants to say his goodbyes to her, and to suss out his sudden urge to sit shiva in respect for her Jewish faith and practice. He wants to grieve the loss of his parent and mentor and to gather his wits and think of the future.

Abruptly, she opens her eyes and insists weakly but wildly, "Take your brother with you!"

"I will."

She relaxes again and says, eyes alight with love, "I knew I could count on you, my dearest boy." She smiles at this tender reference to his childhood, and closes her eyes.

He sits with her, holding her hand. He fills with her light and love as the room dims, as murmuring voices pass and then cease. He starts, realizing that the light has gone out of her: Only her flesh remains. He kisses her forehead and whispers his love, then leaves the hospice to head east on the track to the comm tower. He feels oddly leaden; movement is difficult. Everything looks vivid, clear, final. He looks north across the snow-striped furrows of the fields to the tall poplar windbreaks, beyond which the setting sun backlights thin stratus clouds.

Aaron nears the comm tower, which looks like a lighthouse moored in the woods in the middle of a pasture. When he enters the salvaged metal door, he sees chaos rather than orderly clutter in the accumulation of gizmos and parts, and loneliness rather than solitude in the narrow-curtained bunk and single easy chair. The repurposed paneling looks shabby rather than homey, and adds to the impression that he has been living in an antique electronics shop. He didn't create a timeless life of spirit like that which permeates the community around him; he lived here like a packrat and a loner.

He looks at the breadbox and remembers how his mother would try to persuade him to have a little bread and butter or perhaps buttermilk—or a cup of tea. But she has gone and taken his appetite with her. Right now, those on hospice duty will be washing her body and wrapping it in the winding sheet in preparation for laying her in the ground. They may even wrap Mr. Jensen before the night is out; that worthy has been sleeping for days, wincing and grimacing on his bumpier way to the final rest.

Aaron climbs the spiral stair to the comm room, trying to ignore the profusion of metal, mineral, plastic, and fiber objects that beg repurposing, or the solar water core that runs all the way from beneath the ground floor to the top spire, warming the ground floor, the repair shop, the comm room, and his sleeping quarters under the roof. He looks out through the tall, narrow, water-filled windows that face the four directions; pauses to whisper to the stars; and flips a wide switch to turn on all of the devices, most of which he made from salvaged materials. Transmissions begin to download from all sources, including the biocomm networks—signals from the body of the cosmos and the biome that come in through human communicators and adepts who embody and upload them. As more and more humans receive and share signals generated by life and its context, Aaron wonders whether to bring in a biocommunicator who can take his place and decommission his obsolete technology.

Making a circuit of the comm room, Aaron finds no message that requires a response. This affirms his decision to leave the Amana Colonies without a communicator for the while. Any doctor who wishes to send or to receive messages can contact Aaron—or travel to the communicator in Iowa City or in Ames; something that is unlikely to happen now that doctors have recognized the reams of raw data for what they are: raw bits and bytes that confuse more than they clarify.

Knocking on the ground floor door interrupts Aaron's reverie, and he drops his head. It must be John. While Aaron does not want to be rude to someone who so obviously loved his mother, he cannot face the stranger now. Aaron goes up the folding ladder, eyes on the upstairs bunk where he will shortly lay down but not sleep.

Later, as the shocks of meeting John and agreeing to leave dissipate, he realizes that he is keen to visit Sarah. He will be able to grieve in peace on the journey out, and then spend time with Sarah and Doug, the sole surviving members of his mother's college friendship group. He can also revisit the community where, forty years ago, his mother's story of illness became the basis for a visualization of The Great Poisoning that showed the consequences of modernity so plainly that it altered all their lives. He is proud now of his parents' response, which was the creation of this clinic, and of his own contribution as its first—and only—communicator.

Aaron goes down to the comm room and opens the old armoire where he stores his memory banks. He takes out one that he had in a moment of long-ago whimsy made out of an old toy coin bank and labeled with Sarah's picture. Attaching it to the server, he uses the console he made from old gaming controls to access his mother's calls to Sarah. Glad now that he took the trouble to become a strategic and disciplined archivist, he goes back to 2015 and fast forwards from there, selecting every thousandth frame.

When he reaches 2020, he pauses the record; at this time, he'd seen Sarah as a great beauty. Her hair was blond then, and thick; she still had the posture and tone of a yoga teacher and the fine, almost pinched, symmetric features animated by innate confidence and charisma. That confidence came from the sequence of bold life decisions that took her from a secure job as a career bureaucrat to a life as a yogi and then to the Saltspring Fertility Center founded by their longtime friends Colette and Randall.

Aaron closes his eyes and tries to recall how Sarah looked when he was a boy, when she came to stay at the Denver house while taking a yoga teacher-training course, and again when she went from her studies in Ithaca to Saltspring Island in the Salish Sea near Seattle. Sarah had always been curious and fun-loving; she had shown him how to play in the world. If only he had imbibed her lightness! He resumes his play of 2-D images, watching them age steadily and surely in fast-forward until the screen goes dark. As he flips off the switch, time shock stuns him: Sarah will be gone soon, too, and then he himself will be gone before he has truly lived.

Restlessness grips him. He can't stand to stay put. Tomorrow, hundreds of people will gather to see his mother buried. It will be very public, and he doesn't want to be there. He wants to lock what is left of his family in his heart and go before they bury his living, loving memories. He wants to grieve with Sarah, who is more like family than anyone else alive, and he would not delay their reunion a minute for fear that she may be gone before he gets there. He is even eager to face his estranged brother Eric, who cut himself off from the family when they moved here from Denver. Like their chip-on-the-shoulder father, Eric thought he had a right to their childhood home and took it without a second thought.

Aaron writes a quick note, gathers his gear, locks up the comm tower, and goes to leave his note and keys at the clinic reception desk. Then he crosses the field to Old Man Menno's farmhouse to buy the palomino quarter horse the man has been trying to sell.

2

Damage

Rafaela is standing with her mother inside the big oaken door of the old brick house in which she grew up, and which used to belong to her father Eric's parents. She is in her street clothes, the ones she wears when she wants to look genderless. Her hair is pushed up under her cap; her burlap tunic hangs over her bike pants; her lower legs are streaked in greasy dirt; the bike slippers that came from a dumpster are loose on her feet. She pulls her hat down to her nose to hide her face, and slouches to hide her fitness.

On impulse, Rafa turns back and makes one last effort to get through to her mother, to get her to grasp the netherworld of cybercrime in which Rafa has become entangled.

"Ma! They're playing God! They're not even qualified to be the devil! They're robots, and they're turning me and all my friends into tools, and then into nothing!"

"Go to confession, *chiquita*, tell the priest."

Rafa sighs in frustration, and says bitterly, "You mean my father, the Jewish psychologist confessor?"

"You'll find peace when you reconcile with him, and with the church."

"Ma! The city is dying—the whole world is dying—and the priests just watch from the safety of the sacristy!"

"They did what they could. It's time for each of us to do what we can."

"Dad doesn't even care!"

"He cares for the least among us. You wouldn't leave them behind?"

The sunken black eyes in her mother's creased face and worn body gather every loving impulse into a long gaze. "You're a beautiful young woman, Rafa, inside and out, and you're going to do great good in the world when you find the vocation that you can love with all your heart."

Rafa sighs sharply, as she does whenever her mother reminds her of the initation and vocation projects that she has put off because she doesn't know what to do with her life. Her forehead forms a deep omega sign of sorrow. She opens her mouth to confess all to the one she loves most—then habit takes over. Rafa erases her face, breathes deeply, and resolves to protect her faithful but foolish mother and the surly, sour father who leaves her to her mother while he counsels addicts who go from bad to worse. If his generation had done the real work of change, hers would not have to clean up the mess that humans have been making since Lucy left Africa.

Rafa gives her mother a staccato kiss on the cheek that is equal parts angry desperation and tender care. She then grabs her messenger bag and runs out of the front door of the family home, stuffing into the bag the community college uniform she will put on after she and Mitzi do what they can to set things right. If they fail, they will join their dearest friends beyond the point of no return.

She opens the garage and hops on the street bike that Roberto made for her before devices lured his mind into war-games, biohacking, and finally triggering shootings in distant places.

The vigilantes that lived on ninja fantasies deleted him from life, but they came too slowly; he had become what he hated and spread hell before he died. Rafa and Mitzi tried to pray for him, but transmissions of all kinds were jamming prayer space with noise that stopped love and polluted blessing.

She now realizes with a pang that the only good thing Roberto left behind is the very bike she is riding. The rest is anathema, best forgotten.

Rafa speeds west on the boulevard, dodging bikes, putneys, and carts pulled by diapered horses and oxen. At Colorado Boulevard, she hops the curb and cuts through a city park, gaining speed until her coarse chestnut hair falls into her slipstream, her eyes tear, and her nasal passages desiccate in the desert-dry air. She has gone this way so many times that she hardly notices the zoo-turned-hostel, or the stately capitol turned high security vault, or the old convention and shopping centers turned into shady swap meets and vice marts that would have disgusted the unsinkable Molly Brown.

Beyond those shadowed places, Rafa slows to take heart from the outdoor farm and artisan markets that offer wholesome signs of life during the day. She suppresses the urge to hide in a farm cart and beg for work in the country: Mitzi is waiting. Rafa mustn't be late. She comes up Larimer into the old brick town that has become the hidden hive of Denver's hacking market—and the true engine of its tax-free economy.

The place draws youth from miles around—and idle minds from across the globe—through addictive, all-consuming fantasies that blot out purposeless day jobs. Rafa and Mitzi and their friends once dreamed here and became lost in the narcosis of virtual reality. For the two who remain, their only real choice is to remember Hiroshima and genocide and the Cold War and all the death wishes that pushed life to the edge of extinction. These push them to serve life while their elders cling to the past and spend their future.

Riding down the street, Rafa looks up and around to be sure the four zip lines and twelve ropes are set in the usual way for their messenger route. She worked it up, Scheherazade-like, to serve and amuse Hacker; it bypassed the comm net, distracted and confused outsiders, and reminded him of a cartoon come to life. That amusement bought him time that is fast running out. Fortunately, his arrogance blinds him to the risks that he runs, posed by those who do not share his warped worldview.

Satisfied with the ropes course, Rafa makes a circuit of the nearby streets and alleys, and finally hoists her bike onto an old folding metal stair at the far corner where it will be safe until she releases it from above. Seeing Mitzi's bike on the stair opposite, Rafa stifles the impulse to run; it is too late, and she has nowhere to go.

Taking a deep breath to calm her tremulous limbs, Rafa ascends the stairs, and at the top stops to remove a coil of rope from her pack and to secure it on the landing. She takes hold of it with one hand, aware that her light frame is her greatest advantage, and takes a moment to allow her energy to rise and her senses to sharpen. She smells the manure sitting in the canvas sling beneath the white horse that is Hacker's favorite new toy, the horse that is shying and straining below her on the street with each slam of a metal door or gate.

Rafa strains her ears and thinks she may hear the snap of Mitzi crunching one of the pretzel sticks she likes to bake, and feels a surge of panic that she may never again be annoyed by that sound. Rafa uses that surge to launch herself off the railing, swing to the opposite stair, and deftly grasp a rung of the roof ladder. She gracefully and quietly ascends and propels her body over the fine brick trim onto the metal grate and resin paper roofing. Mitzi is sitting behind the top of the facade, staring at Rafa. She scrambles over and sits down, and Mitzi rests her head on Rafa's lap. Though Mitzi is older, Rafa always plays the role of big sister. They often sit here together watching the street when Mitzi's shift ends and Rafa's begins. Here they must stay until Hacker goes, probably in an hour or so, according to the rhythms of the electronics with which he joined long ago.

The sun rises behind Aaron and his horse, Sleipnir, and turns the Platte River track on which they are walking from a gray and featureless expanse into hardpan etched with ruts and prints. On both sides of the westward track, dew-dotted leaves of grass extend until something stops them. On the left, where spring wildflowers rise above the matted remains of last year's grass, it is the riverbank. The water itself is cloaked by thick white mist. Above, the deep blue sea of air is capped by waves of peach-tinged mare's tails. Ahead stretch the hard-edged shadows of man and horse.

Here on these plains, the sky draws Aaron's mind upward as if in search of something, and Sleipnir's eyes to the ground in search of nourishing tidbits. Here it often seems to the man that they are walking in place. Back on the prairie, he could mark their progress by the subtle watersheds that hold agricultural reserves; the restored Eden lands that need no human care; and the hazardous barrens ringed in barbed wire and marked with chemical, physical, or biological warnings. Here, he sees only the aridity caused by poisoning of the aquifer and abandonment of the land.

Aaron pats Sleipner's neck affectionately and rests his hand there to share warmth. She snorts and nuzzles his shoulder. She seems, at times, to be mothering him; perhaps she remembers teaching him to ride. She is a fatalist and yet a hard worker, and he tries to ease her burden by walking by her side and by finding her treats. Tomorrow they will reach Grand Island and transfer to the wind barge that will take them all the way to Fort Morgan, from where they can walk to Aaron's childhood home in Denver.

The memories that Aaron has been forming since his mother's death rise and possess him. His eyes sink to the trail. His companion becomes skittish as she feels him descend into fitful brooding. In all his years of monitoring the world outside of the Amanas, nothing prepared him for the gap between the comm world—the virtual reality in which he practiced his vocation—and the chaos and confusion of the real world.

That real world is still transiting from fatal modern centralization to the localist, bio-centric, experimental effort to rescue life on earth from human folly. Since leaving the Amanas, every place he has seen has been a patchwork of habitat destruction and rapid restoration. He sees that the modified agricultural habitat of his home is so unusual as to lie outside of the emergence of the Age of Life in Time, as Sarah calls this perilous era. He hopes that her community is at the cutting edge of restoration, as his mother had believed.

He is still amazed, amused, and uprooted by his encounters with the communicators with whom he has been meeting for years in the shared virtual reality of their comm towers. He had not realized how poorly the story of his life fit reality. The task of reinterpreting his past is as large as the one he faced when they moved to the Amanas. He is lucky that he learned personal transformation at his mother's knee and that he is able to process his recent adventures at a good pace.

He returns to his half-cooked memories of Grinnell College. There, he had arranged to carry bark samples from the college to the bioregional lab at Grand Island. In exchange, he received a pass to ride on a barge carrying species up the river to replenish the area around Fort Morgan. While he was in Grinnell, he had gone to see Squill, whose whimsical name and tangential humor had always refreshed Aaron's mood. To his surprise, the real Squill was not at all as Aaron had imagined. After he'd knocked on the door of the comm center west of the campus, the door opened to frame a man in a helmet covered with odd contrivances. Aaron grinned, extended his hand, and said, "You look like you're planning a spacewalk." Squill stood gray-stubbled, withered, and distracted, frozen in mid-movement, muttering and frowning, his neck extended with eyes bugging out in the direction of the ceiling.

"Squill?"

"Not now."

The door shut with a quick click of the lock and would not open again. Aaron lingered, expecting that Squill was joking.

Unwilling to give up easily, Aaron returned three times with the same result before asking about Squill at the college comm center. He learned from a communicator there that Squill had almost died several times from process addictions that made him anorexic. A carer from the old modern clinic went out daily to help Squill eat, wash and dress, and try the latest interventions. This had been Aaron's first vertiginous look into the deep chasm between reality and virtual reality that had claimed so many lives while he was in the bucolic idyll of the Amanas. He would have to rewrite a chunk of his personal narrative just to incorporate it.

A similar set of memories to which his mind keeps returning

concern a woman in the abandoned town of McClellan who had—for fifteen years at least—been sharing her wishful thinking about the town as if it were fact. Her comm center had turned out to be the only remaining venture in town; she had post-dated images from an old collection of photos and reposted new ones from nearby towns. Aaron had admired her gardens, and shared what remained of his provisions rather than partake of her meager store of food. He left with the impression that she could not perceive the gap between her fantasy world and her reality.

In Council Bluffs, he met a communicator with the opposite misperception: his virtual reality was a projection of a dark fantasy. Django, a tattooed, bearded young man who shaved his head and eyebrows and always asked about job leads, had complained that his town was too stingy to support him. He had asked Aaron about job openings for a decade, and Aaron had done many a clever search on Django's behalf. When Aaron got to Council Bluffs, though, he found the city booming and blooming with decorative permaculture in the midst of an unexpected Eden wood. Django worked in a community marketplace reminiscent of a modern crystal palace, except that it generated energy and was dotted with amusements like climbing niches, a waterslide, and a wisdom exchange that was real rather than virtual. There, Aaron earned a sweet store of credits by sharing his real experiences with others who valued them and might put them to good use. Aaron wished he could have stayed with Django or even taken his place.

Sleipnir snorts lightly. Aaron realizes that he has been absently staring at his shadow, watching it shrink. Looking about, he spots an old industrial plant on their right. He has a landmark now by which to measure his progress. As it grows nearer and larger, he can see that it has been stripped for salvage, and is probably abandoned. He cannot tell how old it is, but guesses from the dead walls and its jangling disregard of context that it was built after the decline of industrialism and before the emergence of restoration and renewal.

Aaron hears faint screams approaching the river from the direction of the plant, and spots a land barge coming over a low rise. It has a crew that appears to be a family. Three other land boats follow it over the rise; they are racing. He wonders where they came from: No comm map shows any towns nearby. He wonders if this is a rogue group of insensitives who have taken over a poison barren. The scene seems to be too wholesome for that, but not all insensitives are lawless.

Aaron realizes too late that he hears no crickets chirping, no birdsong welcoming the day. Sleipnir has not swatted a fly for an hour at least. At the riverside there are no dragonflies, no fish sign, no mosquitoes. The grass nearby is stunted and mute. They have been traversing an unmarked poison barren—and there is nothing to be done about that now but to accept whatever fate decides.

Recognizing this, Aaron's mind unfreezes and probes the cause and nature of the barren. He is confused by this singularity; it, too, is out of place in his personal narrative. Was this the result of a production process set in motion with no thought to the consequences? Science gangsterism? Hapless fatalistic, incompetent, or slothful emissions? Or has the kindred of insensitives made the best of an experiment gone wrong? He cannot guess if the hazard is chemical or physical or biological. As he considers these unanswerable questions, he feels more and more befuddled and distressed. When Sleipnir neighs and prods his back, he realizes that fear has gripped him. He must regain his calm for her sake; she depends on him, and he has let her down. She, too, has been breathing and eating the dust in the barren, drinking the water.

"We have to go now," he says to her. He takes her reins authoritatively and guides her forward, his free hand on the crown of the broad-rimmed Amish hat that Old Man Menno gave Aaron as a parting gift, in memory of his mother.

Aaron will have to monitor his body. He has done this for patients who had been in barrens and had come to the clinic for help, patients who sometimes died there. He will monitor his companion, too. He knows all the labs and can read bodily fluids, cells, and DNA himself. His tension eases: He knows what to do. Sleipnir's breathing calms. Soon, she prods him again, and he notices a woman sitting beside the trail on an old brick bench by a stand of trees.

Seeing that she is frail and wasted, he approaches her to offer food. Sleipnir resists. Aaron stops and calls, "Hello?" He examines her face, which is lost in folds like those of a bulldog and lit by hollow, haunted eyes. She does not respond; she is dead to him. Looking at her, Aaron realizes that he too may end this way. It may be days or months—or years—before he knows. He pulls his neckerchief up to cover his nose and mouth and mounts Sleipnir; soon they are both easing their pent-up feelings by galloping away from the rising sun.

3

Courage

M itzi says, "It must have been an hour by now!"
Rafa replies, "No, my sister-friend. Ten minutes."

"Tell me a story," Mitzi says. Her head is heavy on Rafa's thigh.

Rafa looks tenderly at Mitzi, whose growth was stunted by competitive gymnastics imposed by gambling parents. Mitzi, too, has indigenous blood; her skin is dark amber, her hair now dyed bright blue, and her eyes the color of fallen leaves. Mitzi thinks that she is the mirror image of Rafa, but Rafa is slender, her nose aquiline; she is a head taller, and her chestnut hair and maple syrup skin are redder and rougher.

"A story!" Mitzi repeats, her shoulders tight and her neck muscles taut.

"Our story."

"From the start."

"What if we don't have time to finish?"

"Then our story will finish us."

Rafa smiles. No reality fazes her friend. Mitzi is strength and courage; Rafa is comfort and capability.

"After dressing for success, Denver gorged and purged on things; after Hacker defused the robot wars of Arizona, disarmed the missiles of Texas, and finally lost his last footing in real life; after the gurus and masters and revivalists traded their pipe dreams for metal and plastic; after oil and war went to die in

Afghanistan and central Asia; and after modernity crumbled; our land was as it was in 1700. We were dreamers and lovers of God, then, and miscreants and patriots and poor who, like our forefathers, lived in and with the forest."

"After we were born," Mitzi adds, like a child listening to her mother read a favorite book and prompting her when she is slow. "After the twelve of us became friends, and before we became addicted to devices that coopted our story."

"We were not alone, or lonely, or forgotten, or thrown away."

"Or neglected or abused."

"We loved each other with all our hearts." Rafa skips a beat. She doubts this, it is a fantasy and a false promise, a life lesson unlearned—but it is a potent wish, a better narrative than reality can provide. "And then things went wrong, and we lost them. Do you want me to tell you how each of them died?"

"Just say their names, and pause like a funeral bell so we can picture them and say goodbye inside."

Even this may be too much for Rafa, but this is not the time to lose heart. She decides to say each name, and to leave a long pause that gives her time to remember why the two of them are here. She leans back on her palms so that the rough cold metal of the grate steadies her, and the sun rising over the roof edge throws the shadow of her tousled hair onto a window.

Six windows away, Hacker is sitting deep inside a shielded room, unaware that the devices there with him are poisoning his mind. She sighs deeply. Her own desperation drove her into this portentous situation. She will not allow their friends to have died in vain, and so she begins the heart-wrenching litany of those who forgot the cautionary tales of the human past.

"Roberto. Thou shalt not kill." She sees his high cheekbones and golden skin, and Mitzi's lovelorn longing for him. He seemed the best but fell first, fastest, and farthest.

"Cash," says Mitzi.

"Remember the Sabbath, and keep it holy."

"What was his Catholic name?"

"I don't know." When Rafa sees Cash in her mind's eye, he looks colorless; only his deep, shiny red hair and eyebrows show color. He was a stranger to sun and fresh air, and a slave to his namesake. He worked non-stop, joining them now and then between jobs until he got one that took all his time and still failed to fend off the storm of bills that besieged his single mother and sibs. When his absentee boss replaced him with a device, he went to Colorado Springs and was shipped to a far-off country where not even his corpse would rest in peace for a day—or for eternity.

"Teresa."

"Thou shalt not curse."

"You changed it!"

"I called it. She didn't use holy names when she cursed, but it killed her all the same."

Mitzi heaves a ragged sigh. "True."

Rafa wants to say more—much more—but she leaves it at that. There is no point in being angry at the dead; that is cursing, too. The best way to remember Teresa is to bless her beginning. When she came to them with Cash, she'd had the color he lacked. She was ebony, slender as a cornstalk with a black tassel, bowed over by a slouch that hid her height. She was nocturnal like Cash—and, with time, the others. When Cash died, she'd turned to ginga, the black magic of her native Brazil, and turned her grief into hateful cursing. In the end, she craved death and the sixth extinction that most Denverites see as unavoidable. Her rage-filled form finally exploded in a bloody, mutilating fight that mangled her flesh.

"Paolo."

"Thou shalt not lust," Rafa says tensely.

"Say it the old way! I'm too scared to say something I've done."

"I'm scared too. You say it your way and I'll say it mine?"

Mitzi pinches a fold in Rafa's burlap tunic and says, "Thou shalt not commit adultery."

"Paolo did both," Rafa says. She is still disgusted with the slight and sensual Paolo, who seemed to think he had something to prove. He was Sicilian and a throwback and knew full well what might happen to his family when he bedded his married cousin and, in time, each of her sisters. Rafa can't imagine what they had seen in that calculating clown of a boy. They must have yielded to angry despair, and provoked their detested husbands to dispatch them to old-fashioned, open-casket funerals with burials in sanctified ground.

Rafa shifts her seat so that she can see between the crenellations of the old brick facade, and watch the iron door that has not has yet sent out its signature sound, the one that begins her day as a messenger. She takes off her cap and tunic, revealing her acrobatic leotard.

"Ceecee."

"Thou shalt have no other Gods before me."

"Because I am a jealous God. But can God be jealous of devilry?"

"I'd say she put God second—and then last."

"You're just making our litany fit the Ten Commandments!"

Mitzi's fear is getting the better of her; she doesn't usually take it out on Rafa. Rafa strokes her hair kindly. "I don't think so."

"Maybe it was meant to be like this. Maybe we'll live."

"Maybe. Or maybe my dad's right and there is no God."

"There is. It's just that we're like Ceecee: In over our heads."

"Doing our best."

"I hope it's good enough."

"Are we ready for a time of trial?"

"Let's pray to be." Mitzi closes her eyes.

Rafa watches the brown-painted iron door behind which so much evil has taken place. She prays, distractedly, that they will not be enraptured by the forces of destruction in the way that Ceecee was beguiled by the siren cycle of sin and saving. Rafa had barged in on Cash and Ceecee once when they were caught in an abject agony of humiliation that they then followed up with the heady ecstasy of union. Ceecee was always tense then, always ready to fly up to the glittering peak of triumph and down to the loathsome pit of abject self-abasement, always returning to the engine of exciting exorcism that propelled the highs that ended in lows. Soon Hacker, too, was enthralled with her, and when Cash left, took time away from his accustomed electronic addictions to bed Ceecee and shift her addictions to online gaming and gambling. She, too, disappeared—and turned up in a closed casket. Rafa does not even want to guess what happened, and neither does the parish whose careless loss of youth has nearly awakened it to care of creation. Now only she and Mitzi seem aware of how badly they are all missing the mark.

"Cartoon," Mitzi continues.

"Thou shalt not covet."

"I wish somebody had something I wanted!"

Rafa smiles, then laughs at their pain. "You want to be tempted?"

"I want to want something."

"You want the only thing that matters—life and all its possibilities. If we live, we'll be bathed in it and belong to it."

"We'll be part of something with no big ego, and no blindness to right and wrong."

"Maybe we'll find each other."

"No! They'd find us if we did!"

Rafa sighs. She thinks of Cartoon's mother who was always at work, and who left him to raise himself with the help of cartoons. Rafa went with Cartoon to the factory where his mother worked, and saw the punch press to which she was chained. In went her hands to position a flat piece of metal; out they came again, pulled by chains that preserved her fingers; down crashed the press; and back in went her hands to pull the punched piece away and to put another in. She earned just enough to buy the merch to go with her son's cartoons, and had just enough time to take pleasure in his ephemeral joy.

He was everything to her, and he took her for granted, thinking it only natural that her hands would move all night in her sleep as if she were part of a machine. He also took in her desire; he wanted little more than to delight, briefly as a crow, in new and shiny objects. When she died—alone as he had been alone—he had taken to staring into the shop windows in the marketplaces, and to taking small items from friends. Unsatisfied and mad with desire, he took a baseball bat and perpetrated a crystal night of broken windows, during which a frightened night watchman shot him dead. Neither Rafa nor Mitzi had gone to that funeral; they could no longer abide passive fatalism or helpless frustration. They began to try their wits and wiles against their death-bound world.

"What about your Ma?" Mitzi asks.

"What about her? She cares, but she's afraid of everything. She can't help me,"

"I feel bad about mine. She's so helpless. I'm never having kids."

Rafa smiles. Mitzi is wired and optimistic; if she lives, she is likely to change her mind.

"Hash. Honor thy father and thy mother."

"And do what they say, not what they do."

"We'll do what we do for them, too," Mitzi says, looking up to meet Rafa's eyes. "For Hash."

Rafa nods. She pictures Hash with all the others, standing like ten pins, looking their best, and blesses them. As if the blessing had rebounded as living, loving light she, too, is blessed by love and gratitude for their brief lives. She is filled with steely resolution to live the best life she can for them, through the coming danger and into the distant future. She sees Hash as she was, big in every way, her triple D bra size distracting all eyes from the rolls of fat lined up below like an upside-down stacking toy. She had been calm and easygoing and seemed to be the one who could hear all their troubles unmoved. But soon she was smoking and selling basement weed, and then hash and bhang, and attracted a small-time crime pimp called Cook who designed drugs and then tried them on her. When her parents tried to stop her, she planted drugs in their home and called the SWAT team. They were taken away and put in prison, where a prisoner who hated Cook killed them; Cook, seeing her state, had given her more and more downers that finally took her down beneath the ground.

"C.T."

"Thou shalt not bear false witness."

Rafa squirms to think of C.T.'s betrayal of her parents. The ten had all been neglected and abused in one way or another, but none had taken it so badly or responded so vindictively as C.T. She, too, had Native blood, and knew that her mother had prayed to the Earth Goddess for conception. With innuendo and sly denunciation, she had persuaded the church to bar her parents, who then came apart slowly before her eyes and finally left town. On the way south, her father drank and drove the horses too hard. Their cart overturned and crushed them and all their children.

Rafa and Mitzi had tried to reason with the other friends who remained, but the effort had come too late: They had drawn the interest of Hacker. He had especially liked Francie, who seemed frail but was strong in hidden places.

"Francie," Mitzi says, a lump in her throat. If they are not careful, they will lose heart. "I wish we could start!"

"This is when it's hardest. Time is our medium, and we can't work against it."

Mitzi sits up, looks at her breathlessly, and lies down again. "You're right."

"Let's think of Francie." Francie had ignored Hacker and returned blessings for curses. For a time, she had seemed to awaken his deeply-buried best self, but then his group of bio hackers, now wired together to form a group mind, had hacked her and gotten her to steal rare metals and precious custom-made circuits from rival groups; those rivals had soon disposed of her.

"Belinda," Mitzi says, tears running across her face, sobs seizing her breath. "Beautiful, beloved Belinda. I loved Roberto, and then her, and now you. You know that, don't you? I wouldn't want us to die without—without…"

"Yes I know, and I love you like my twin sister. I hope that's enough."

"You do? You don't just love me 'cause I'm the only one still alive?"

"We kept each other alive through love. We can't stop now."

"Bad timing, that'd be bad timing," Mitzi laughs. "I wish—I wish we had kept her alive."

"We couldn't. She was too beautiful, too good a target."

Rafa sees Belinda's hazel eyes, black hair, and freckled skin. Her short dreads made a jet-black halo around her radiant smile, and her soft, thin skin made her collarbones and hands stand out. She had a touch of Spanish on her tongue, and her melodious voice could enchant them with any gospel song right up until Hacker got a smack-stricken neurosurgeon to put an implant in her temple. She had wasted away in front of their horrified eyes, and turned them into avenging angels.

As the barge moves away from the docks, Aaron grooms the exhausted Sleipnir, who is resting uneasily in a narrow stall. When she is calm, he explores the cargo lashed to the deck, wending his way between crates of nesting or newborn animals; shelves stacked with starts of tenacious seeds; aquaculture tanks full of hatchling fish; phials of amphipods; and racks of wood-hived insects. After that, like an Odin-Noah, he fathers the young and hopeful habitat restorers as they wait to play Johnny Appleseed to habitats long neglected or abused. He shares their pleasure when the wind barge passes buffalo herds dining on sweet grass. These passengers know that the herds' leavings are fertilizing the soil and thus refreshing the microbiomes of all species living the length and breadth of the range.

Confined by the barge, they soon grow restive and release energy in music and dances. Aaron soaks up their high spirits. The next day, when they hear his story, they express sorrow and make a minyan with him so that he can properly say the mourner's Kaddish for his mother, and again for each dead swath of sand and rock and badly-stunted grass that they pass. From time to time the barge stops and some disembark, unfold and load their pull carts, and follow compass settings like evangelists of the new good news, their faith in life and love shining like ever-burning bushes in the wilderness. One by one he blesses them and wishes them well on their way.

At the final stop of Fort Morgan, Aaron and Sleipnir debark and walk out on a sand bar. Alone again, horse and man stretch and stumble, feeling their way back into their stride and their strength. Whitman-like, they seek divine love in the busy town. Behind them, the mules and wind barges that mark the river's course recede with the musky smell of animals and the savory smoke of riverside peace pipe cafes. They skirt the bazaar, looking for a place to stable Sleipnir so that Aaron can replenish their stocks of dried oats and barley, dried vegetables and fruit, and the goat cheese for which Fort Morgan is known. Later, laden down with food, he finds his companion again and pauses to enjoy the old Colorado brick town hall, now surrounded by the rammed-earth sanctuaries of the New Exodus movements that welcome all who love life.

He spies a skyward flash of light and, excited, tells Sleipnir, whose eyes fill with ennui, of the fliers held aloft by sun and air. He has not seen an airplane for many a year, and watches with delight as a flight of ultralights fans out like a blooming chrysanthemum, carrying provisions and news and medical aid to the buffalo and to their human caretakers. He has heard and still believes that this fleet is catalyzing the ongoing restoration of the plains. Without it, this region of earth might be like so many others, sickened by human hands and then left to fate. Aaron turns his attention to this fleet and to the many other signs of resilience and transformation that he has seen and taken to heart. He can use the bad as priming for the good, and the good to strengthen his faith and courage in life.

During the long ride to Denver, Aaron looks ahead across the land and uses that perspective to sustain his spirits all the way to the city's outskirts. There, he stops his companion and they both take some water. He lingers to acknowledge that he would prefer to go without seeing his bitter brother. He had thought himself equal to returning to the city of his childhood. He had tracked its stasis and decline, watched it fail to emerge from what his mother called the black hole at the end of modernity. She had never forgiven the city. Even while knowing it to be a lifeless thing, she had held a grudge against it for trying just once and then giving up, for desecrating its remaining life. She had worried ceaselessly about Eric, too, until she finally gave up on him and made her peace with his choices. She had held the family's ground while his father came round as well as he could, and while Aaron created a good—if sterile—life. Now both she and his father are gone, and the mending of the familial rift with Eric has come down to Aaron.

Despite his attempts to prepare himself for this, as Aaron feels the old, too-tall, too-intense comm towers loom, they crush his spirit. He contracts. His interbeing—the intangible entangling envelope of his body—pulls inward like the soft tentacles of a sea anemone. He is enervated and depressed. Sleipnir becomes balky, and Aaron places a protective net over himself and his companion. They leave the track, find a campsite, and sleep fitfully inside their veils. Aaron speaks softly to his companion in hopes of sustaining their equipoise long enough to embrace his brother, perhaps for the last time.

The next morning, they draw nearer to the spectacular

foothills of the Rockies that rise from the wide valley of the Platte. The sinister modern skyline cuts across the scene like rubble strewn by a catastrophe too slow and too big to be noticed. They head resolutely toward it, reaching the streets at twilight. The solar street lamps switch on to reveal slum buildings beside old asphalt roads. These are brightened by the fraying burlap bags of hanging gardens, and by arrays of vertical membrane windmills standing idle in the still air of evening, air that smells of charcoal and rubbish fires. Aaron pulls his thick neckerchief up over his nose and mouth and tucks it in his collar. He sees tags on the walls and realizes that he is in a lawless area, or, rather, an area where chaos is suppressed by violence. The decay is orderly, though. Perhaps Denverites prefer tyranny to unpredictable trouble.

As they progress into Denver, Aaron walks backward through his life all the way to the empty streets of the old inner city. Now, though, instead of seeing dark interiors lit by television tubes, he sees glowing comm streams and VR props that hold their human quarry in place for days at a time.

His heart is heavy with sorrow. He worries, briefly, that something here will set off a poison in his flesh, and then deliberately turns his heart forward to Sarah. Soon they have arrived in the old streets where once-grand homes like his parents' have been preserved as hives for ventures or homes for groups. His heart warms to this evidence of social evolution, this sign that some here have not lost heart. He begins to spot shadows coming and going in the moonlight, and finds the air clean enough to let down his neckerchief and doff his hat to strangers.

"Hello, friend," says a young woman who passes on the sidewalk with a flick of a long braid over black sackcloth. He has reached the neighborhood of the New Universal Friends. He soon loses his way, and stops to ask directions of another Friend with an unexpected ear curl who stops to ask about Aaron's old-order hat. After a polite exchange of pleasantries, the Friend says that he knows Eric and offers condolences for the alcoholism that has overtaken him. The man says a blessing on the death of a mother and leaves Aaron speechless. He does not know if he is more surprised by the encounter, or by the man's knowledge of him and Eric.

Continuing on, Aaron enters the boulevard on 17th Street and sees City Park ahead, just as it was decades ago. There on the left is his old brick home, its trim still green, now with a windmill atop the upstairs turret and another along the roofline. Eric has kept some pride of place, but the gall-infested spruce is still there—and still infested. Sleipnir nickers. She knows, somehow, that they have arrived.

Aaron releases her reins and walks up to the door slowly, a riot of conflicting feelings swirling in his core. Pulling himself together, he knocks, perhaps too loudly.

There is a stirring upstairs in his old room, the billowing of a curtain, a rush of footsteps on the stairs. The door swings wide and a tiny figure squeezes his breath away. Her voice whispers, "You must find Rafa at Black Lake and take her with you!"

After Rafa's voice dies away, and Mitzi is less stressed by the delay, she asks thoughtfully, "What about our sin?"

"We didn't lie. We said we would be his messengers and we were. We're not going to steal. We're going to snatch and destroy illegal devices. We're doing it to protect others. We're doing it for the ten who went down unprotected by the oldest warnings against the best-known mistakes."

The iron door bangs and reverberates; Rafa and Mitzi startle.

Rafa peers over the roof edge with an intense gaze. Time was, Hacker would have sensed her and clocked her without looking; now, he is oblivious to living systems. His broadband mind is dispersed in all directions, fully absorbed but never focused, never wholly human. He is everywhere and nowhere, a thing of things, a tool of tools. In a moment, he slides down the rope she put up for him and disappears into the alley beside his virtual grotto.

Rafa and Mitzi toss their bags near their bikes, grip the roof edge, vault gracefully onto the ledge below, and grasp the rope ends hooked beside them. Drawing those ends behind them like an open belt, they hold on tightly and swing in tandem across the street, alighting on the top landing of the fire escape opposite. They hear a smattering of applause and recall that they have become something of a marketing tool that both conceals and reveals what goes on within, like in the old days of Prohibition.

Rafa and Mitzi secure the ropes. As Rafa enters through the iron door, Mitzi mounts the rail and delights the small crowd with an improvised routine of hand balancing and acro dancing. Inside the loyalist party room, beyond the steampunk gaming and craft stations and colorful arrays of moonshine, stands the door to an inner room of floor-to-ceiling electronics. At this hour, the door is open; in the doorway, on a salvaged 100-year-old stool, sits Bot, who raises his eyebrows slightly to acknowledge her.

"What do you have for me?"

"On the desk. Ten pieces. More in an hour."

"Right."

They hear a scream outside. Mitzi is either pretending to fall or—if the trick didn't work—has actually fallen. Rafa may never know. From this point, they will head in different directions. If all goes as planned, they will rendezvous south of the sand line at the toilet in the diesel station outside the biggest solar array east of the Continental Divide. Rafa swallows her fear. Bot, who is not as far gone into process addictions, reads her fear and rushes out.

In his absence, she darts to the outbox that dangles from the ceiling. It is an old, used rural mailbox that was bashed in by a baseball bat at some point in its checkered past. From it, Rafa snatches the messages and scoops out the rare and costly implants crafted in the sterile room on the floor below, the implants she will destroy so that they cannot ruin any more of Hacker's targets. Dropping the stash of pockmarked stainless cylinders into her bra pocket, she rushes out to find Bot and Mitzi. She is curiously concerned about Bot, who did not consent to the scheme but may end up its scapegoat, if all goes well. Rushing to the rail where he is standing, Rafa falls against him to make him angry with her, for his own protection; he has a temper. It works briefly, before he is distracted and distressed by the sight of Mitzi lying on the ground, and by the attention her mishap will bring.

"I'd better go!" Rafa says, sending out a prayer that Mitzi's stunt worked, that she's okay. Rafa continues on her route, delivering the messages up and down the streets and alleys of the old town. A small group of spectators and the usual gang of slickly-dressed street children follow her and cheer her shows of skill, or try to hit her with slingshot stones. Today, she is too distracted by the special demands of this, her last circuit, to heed anything but the kinesthetic patterns that carry her from each rooftop, ledge, or staircase to the next.

Soon she has placed each message in its bin or box or slot. Before she is fully aware of having finished and recovered her bike and bags, she has dismounted by the train tracks and is whizzing along a meticulously-planned route through suburban streets where oblivious owners of American dream houses—the error that blotted out so many habitats—dwell with their aging hoards of nothings. Her face and eyes are stinging. Her hair is knotting. She attends to only one thing: the bulge in her bra. She must get it to the Sedalia solar collector or lose all for nothing.

An hour or more later—she is not sure how long—she reaches the diesel station and breaks into the old toilet with ease. She and Mitzi chose it because it is big enough to hold both their bikes, and remote enough that they can leave separately and unseen. They will then make their way from it to the labyrinth of old mine shafts outside of town, where each will find a place to hide and sleep during the day, before setting out to ride 10 or 20 miles closer to a chosen Eden land every night.

Rafa turns on the light and stands at the chipped porcelain sink, looking into the cracked mirror. She combs out her hair, imagining that she is adorning herself for a dance, or preparing to play Pachamamma in a pageant, or sitting down with children all around like a storyteller of old. She would be admired and desired, and would believe that a man could be her match, or even overmatch her. It is her secret wish to desire a man. She would rather pine away in adoration, or claw a response from a reluctant face, than feel nothing for any man.

Rafa washes her body and pulls a close-fitting corset dress from her bag. She is, in an old-timey sleazy way at least, costumed and groomed. To wait for Mitzi without giving way to worry, Rafa decides to do her hair in tiny braids. She has finished the right side of her scalp when she hears the outside doorknob jiggle, and waits breathlessly to see who is there. Mitzi bursts in with her bike, face alight, laughter in her chest. She tackles Rafa with a sweaty embrace. Rafa takes a raggedy sigh and sobs sloppily on Mitzi's shoulder.

"Eeew! Wipe your snot."

Rafa laughs sheepishly. "And you—wash your body. Your stink is making me cry."

Mitzi pulls off her clothes, throws her bike panniers aside, and does a gymnastic move over the sink that lets her use it like a bidet. Rafa looks away and listens as Mitzi crows about her stunt, the soft fall that fooled everyone and that bought her a getaway ride which had unfortunately taken her in the wrong direction. She'd had to jack a bike from someone speed-training on a nearby trail, and took the time to throw him some silver pellets that she hopes he will know how to use. Rafa slides down the wall and squats against it, allowing herself to release her worry and recover her resolve.

"Rafa. Rafa!"

Mitzi is standing above her, seemingly exultant. "I'm so glad you're safe," she confesses with a gleaming smile and no trace of irony.

"And I you," Rafa says heartfully, "but our energy is all over the place. We can't go in until we focus."

Mitzi squats beside her. "That may not happen. My legs feel like fish fins."

Rafa smiles. "I have accordion arms."

"Okay, let's stand, and eat."

"In here?"

"Where else?"

"I suppose," Rafa says, making a face and then smiling at her ill-timed fastidiousness. They pull out snacks and devour them purposefully, brush their teeth, and set off on foot for the control center of the array. The sandy ground has been stabilized by invasive grasses that do much less to restore the earth's skin than do the bio-crusts to the east and west. It is not too hot or too dry here now, in the nocturnal hours when the Milky Way is strewn above and the bats, undeterred by acres of radially-arrayed reflective panels, seek pollen in the flowers that remain. Rafa lags behind a bit to conceal the way she folds her arms over her crown in irrational fear of these flying friends of life.

They knock on the door of the mobile office that houses the lone night sentinel, Chuck, who scans the plant in search of problems that call for early-morning maintenance or repairs. He answers the door promptly. Chuck knows that they have an agenda and has made his peace with that; he is too lonely to object to their visit and too smart to ask why they came. He trusts them to do him no harm. They have been cultivating him for weeks, coddling him, tempting him, wheedling his schedule out of him, discovering the exact place where they can glue the devices down to melt without doing damage so that they will, with luck, disappear from the world.

Rafa puts on some music that Chuck likes. He has been waiting for this, she can tell. As Mitzi disappears, Rafa turns him away from the array and sits across his lap. He must have been thinking of her; it is over in minutes. She stifles a sob, but when he accepts her gift with warm affection she does not mind being kind in this way, and feels that humane joining in this sterile place is a kind of love, an act of nature that is free of lust. He should be safe; it's all on camera, the perfect alibi. When he is finished, she takes his round, bearded face and looks into his pale blue eyes for the first time.

"Remember me," she says. "I will not forget you, or your kindness." Her face contracts in sorrow.

He hugs her, and she is comforted. She hears Mitzi clear her throat.

"I have to go. And I can't come back again. I'm sorry. It's … my parents. They're getting suspicious."

When she sees how bereft he looks, she feels a pang of remorse and says, "When you see the Milky Way, think of us." And then she and Mitzi are running toward the bathroom, dressing for a night ride, and heading over the field to the place from which Mitzi will go up and west and Rafa will go north. They hug, and then Mitzi kisses her passionately. Rafa accepts it with patience and sisterly love and wills their embrace to become a holy kiss.

Later, after Rafa has reached and passed through Central City, she stops to call her mother. When her mother answers, Rafa does not speak. Her mother says, "You may be able to catch your *tío* at the old camping place."

Rafa knows where her mother wants her to go. She rings off, crying, and at the next mine shaft throws her phone into its depths.

4

Rendezvous

Rafa hears him approach her simple camp at Lake Mills, which she has made more comfortable with the goods she cached above Jewel Lake last summer. His is a gentle, tender voice conversing amiably with a clopping, nickering horse. She quickly conceals the trappings of her lakeside camp in the bosky backdrop of the boulder that is hiding her bike. She hops behind that boulder and uses it as a blind. She is worried when the man stops at the foot of the Lake, and hopes that he does not see her hiding place as he looks up the trail to Black Lake, which also accesses Shelf Lake and the spine of the continent.

As the man dismounts near the outlet of the lake and pats his horse, she recognizes him as Aaron, whom she once saw in a photo hidden in Ma's trinket box. He is sandy-haired with gray whiskers that are beginning to form a chevron beard; his broad shoulders and deep chest accentuate his modest height and boney legs. His nose is a right triangle in profile—like hers but with a narrower base—and his mouth and chin are broad and prominent. He looks nothing like her father, though his careful, economical movements suggest the same deliberate character.

When he smiles, relieves his horse of all burdens, and leads her gently to a grassy area on the lakeside, Rafa realizes that Aaron is more like Ma than like her father. He offers love, faith, and care to his animal companion, not the self-pitying sarcasm with which her father escalates blame and offense. She inhales sharply, and her breath catches his ear. He looks her way and then scans and studies the shore of the lake from its head to its foot. She holds her breath.

After a long few minutes, Aaron begins to set up camp. She continues to watch, adjusting her position for comfort. He soon disappears up the trail to gather brush, and then makes a fire on a rocky shelf across from the horse's greensward. She can already tell that the evil that her father spoke of Aaron is a lie. The basis of her life story weakens; she is almost panting with something like fear.

She orients her life to biological time, as embodied in the high forest that is alive and may still recover from the wounds of heat that took half the trees. She sees temperature-resistant seedlings coming in, but they have yet to thrive in this place. As she watches, shy animals who have been watching both Rafa and her uncle from the fragrant subalpine forest resume their activities. A woodpecker pounds a snag on the opposite slope; a dipper hops up the lake shore in front of her, searching for insects; a nervous pica—Rafa wonders if it is the last one—darts up the slope, startling a marmot. Rafa's eye is caught by the flight of a mountain bluebird and by a glimpse of a western tanager in a tree. Soon those birds hide as a curious hawk rides an updraft into the distance, and an owl hoots.

Below them, Aaron crosses his legs and begins to say a prayer in Hebrew, the same one her father said the night that John came and told them that Eric's mother had died. Rafa had never seen a face so altered by shock and regret. She listens to her uncle and thinks lovingly of her friends. She would like to mourn them this way.

He is silent for a time, during which she gathers the courage to approach him—but then he screams abruptly and frightens her foolish. She freezes, and waits. He calls out again. He is remonstrating and mourning in Hebrew. The sound jogs a memory that floats to the surface, a memory of her father mocking his mother's love of Jewish superstitions, like crying out to God in the wilderness. As Aaron cries out again, something glistens equidistant between them. A bear has emerged from the trees that line the stony shore. As the bear's nose delicately samples the air pooled over the lake, Aaron falls silent again, resting his forehead on his hands. The bear withdraws, as if respecting Aaron's sorrow.

When the bear has lumbered away, Rafa rises clumsily and says awkwardly, "Hi!"

Aaron starts and sits up, his silhouette silvered by moonlight. He laughs quietly. "I saw your bike, but I thought that if you were here you'd have come out by now!" As he adds some brush to the fire he asks, "Would you like some sage tea?"

Rafa realizes that she is chilled through. "Yes!"

He looks at her intently. "It's good to finally see you. Your mom wrote and told us about you, from time to time, so I feel like I know you a bit."

Up close, in the firelight, she sees that while he has the form of a young man, nature has sketched age on his skin; it is splotched and sagging around the eyes and neck. She looks shyly away and watches the vapor of her breath disappear. "I didn't know anything about you until just now, when I saw how different you are from Dad. I knew you didn't look like him, but he had nothing but bad things to say about family."

Aaron sighs. "I wish I could say I'm surprised. And I wish I could have seen him. But he was away somewhere."

He brews and pours the tea, handing her a cup. He has few

things, but they seem to be the right ones. She looks away from the firelight long enough to take reassurance from the stone heights graced by the moon's light. "When John came and told Dad that your mom died, Dad said that prayer."

Aaron starts, and then asks in disbelief, "Who is this John? I hadn't seen him since 2010 and suddenly there he was sitting on her deathbed."

"He's a friend of Sarah and Doug. He came to Denver to tell us that your mom died, and that you would be coming."

Aaron frowns. "I didn't know. I didn't expect him." He smiles slyly and adds, "I didn't expect you either, but I'm glad to be here with you, where the family used to hike before Eric went his own way. Strange to see it deserted."

"People who like the wild are gone from Denver. Those who come here follow the elk, and won't be back until the aspen leaves turn gold."

"Are you coming with me?"

"I guess so. Mom told me to come here to find you."

"She said something about trouble," he says gently.

Before Rafa knows what she is doing, her story pours from her lips, along with tears from her eyes, snot from her nose, and sobs from her gut. When she finishes, her head is laying on his knee as Mitzi's had lain on hers, and he is stroking her hair as she had done for her dearest friend. She feels nakedly exposed right down to the core of her long-contracted being, and begins to shiver from cold and fear. He overflows with care. She receives his comfort in the fullness of their silence. Then she is crying again for never having felt such healing love from her father. And then she is talking again, exploring, processing, and working things through, finding a way forward through the wilds that she had cached inside.

Finally, she stops, exhausted. An owl hoots somewhere downstream.

Aaron laughs. "You're just like your grandma. I didn't expect that either."

"How can I be? I never even knew her," asks Rafa plaintively.

"You try to make things right. You take responsibility. I don't know how you got like that, but you did. Your dad is probably more like her than we know. He cares for people Mom and Dad didn't. People time left behind."

Rafa relaxes and draws in a halting sigh.

"I'm sorry you went through all that," Aaron says solemnly. "Fortunately, process addictions die in the wild. You should be safe from addicts here—but we should be cautious. I can check the comm net as we go. I'm a communicator, so I can do that from any place. Mom would have said she was looking out for us, and who knows? Maybe she is."

"Where are we going? Please tell me it isn't Denver. I'm worried about Ma and Mitzi, but…"

"We're headed to Portland to meet Doug. He'll take us by boat to Saltspring."

"Is Portland like Denver?"

"I don't expect so. Denver has a history of boom and bust, of trying once and giving up. When I was small, the windmills and solar panels had been tried and taken away. Portland has a history of self-sufficiency and cooperation and trying and trying again. I hear they made a lot of mistakes—nearly ruined a large part of Cascadia—but kept rebounding and evolving."

"What's it like where you're from?"

"Good. Alive. But patchy, very patchy."

"Scary. But hopeful," Rafa says.

"As of today, you and I will be making a new history for our family, and we'll soon be making one with Sarah's community, something to do with a legacy."

"What's that?"

"I wish I knew. I trust we'll find out from Sarah."

"I feel like a small child. I've always been one, and never been one."

"Then let's eat like adults and sleep like babies."

"I want to do my part to make dinner and such," Rafa insists.

"Sounds like a plan," he says. He waits for her to sit up, then stretches and goes to collect the makings of a meal.

5

Oasis

Aaron lazes in the almost scalding water of the largest hot spring pool at the traveler's spa in Cove, Columbiana. He has spent as much time as possible luxuriating in its cleansing waters since they decided to rest here. Later, they will ride to the dock on the Columbia River in Umatilla and take the wind turbine barge upriver to Portland, where they will meet Doug. Here at Cove they are among pilgrims—mostly New Brethren and retirees—who are traveling a route that begins in a recovering forest to the north, skirts a nuclear barren, and ends in a new Eden land to the south. Aaron and Rafa will stay until they have earned enough credits for the journey ahead by telling stories of their travels.

Tonight he may tell of Riverside, a town in a broad and fertile pasture on the North Platte framed by the Medicine Bow Mountains, through which some traders and herders follow wild bison and wapiti and others stop with their domestic herds. He can see it in his mind's eye, and watch as the clouds reveal streams and eddies of air flowing over the mountains and down into a high valley that is cool and free of wildfires. It reminds him of the Colorado of his youth, before pine beetles and heat presaged the sandline that is traveling north, undoing the restoration of the forests of the continental divide.

As Aaron relaxes into the heat of the pool, his mind wanders to the risks and privations of their long hard ride: the saddle sores, the slow bowing of the thigh bones, the cracking and bleeding of thirsty lips, the rocky ground that disturbed sleep, and the turkey jerky that erased all memory of what it was to live to eat. He enjoyed watching Rafa—who had followed far behind on her bike so as not to spook Sleipnir—become a skilled navigator of damaged lands. He has confidence that she will not wander into hazards as he did: like a naïf exiting a well-loved land.

All of their trials prepared them for the enchantment of this refuge, this oasis in the wilderness that they hope will be the end of hardship. It occurs to him that the other pilgrims' journeys have not been as physically arduous, and that some will have continued in the colonial error of seeing life as something separate from them, as a tool for gaining goods and privilege. They will have missed their previous errors and the chance to recognize the modern sterility of exigeses of ancient scriptures. They will have glossed over the living lessons that make it possible for the lion and lamb in him to lie down together in his heart. Few of the pilgrims Aaron has met have learned from gentle Shakespeare how to turn retribution into reconciliation, or from mystical followers of the golden rule how to turn Torah into beatitudes and nigguns and understanding of the unforgivable. They may shy away from rather than come to terms with the sin of vitacide that nearly extinguished their species along with all others.

To date, Aaron's stories have been too light: He has been inspiring listeners who have no need of him. He has said nothing to those who still see wilderness as "hideous and desolate and full of beasts" rather than full of life, those who are still strangers to the body of life embraced by Thoreau in his consumption and Whitman in his ecstasy of inclusive love. The eyes of such pilgrims' hearts look at the world through states like fear rather than care or cure. He must show them the errors of the ancestors so that they can discover who they would become.

"*Tío, Tío*! Wake up!" Rafa's eyes are big and round. She's sitting on the edge of the spring in her spa towel, flushed and panting with heat. He too is too hot. He lifts himself out of the water and sits beside her.

"I was thinking, not sleeping," Aaron says.

"About what?"

"It's time to tell them about the bad places."

"The barrens?"

"No, they've seen the obvious ones. They've seen several that anyone can tell are bad. We need to show them a penchant for killing that they too know well to see as a fault."

"Like what? A throwback church?"

"No, no. Like a pre-barren, something that was a part of the problem but that still enchants them."

"Won't that make them sadder?"

"If we do it wrong, or they take it wrong. If we do it right and they take it right we'll set them up to do the right thing in their own way, in their own time."

"That's a bit much to expect."

"I may as well try. What's the worst that could result?"

"A lynching?"

Aaron laughs. "They can't burn me at the stake, there's a burn ban."

"That's not funny."

"If I'm afraid, they'll be afraid."

"I need you here."

"And I need you." He enjoys an avuncular smile and tips his head back to look up through the canopy of pines, closing his eyes to the bright sun. "I'm going to cool off in the cold pool and see if it puts me in the mood to tell a tale in verse, like our Viking ancestors."

Rafa looks incredulously at the sky like a child appealing to an absent father, and then laughs her disbelief.

Aaron winks. He is conscious of playing the movie cowboy as he drawls, "I'm glad to know I can still surprise you."

"Still? When do you NOT surprise me?"

Aaron feels smug until a lone jump into the cold pool constricts his privates; then he remembers that he has never written a poem, has no topic yet, and is set to speak in several hours. He leaves the cold pool refreshed, speeds out through the shower area, and enters the wide woods to seek their mute counsel. A few hours later, after he has tried and cast aside ancient meters, has struggled to rhyme, and has lost the thread of his story, he settles for some sense of rhythm that drives his point and then dashes through a late dinner.

Afterwards, he rushes to the tea room where a small crowd has gathered in hopes of putting down the leaden burden of reflecting on their ancestors' errors. He winks at Rafa, who is waiting on stage, and approaches her to jump up, join her, and take up a guitar. He spends a moment looking at each audience member in turn, relaxes deeply, and then smiles and begins casually, "I aimed for poetry with music, but let's just call it a prose poem with punctuation by guitar." He strums and begins.

"An uncle on a horse and a niece on a bike trace the craggy face of a devastated land, the uncle grieving, the niece fleeing;

"Progressing as pilgrims on a blanket of life decimated by a human plague, riding and raising pine-infused dust;

"The elder tastes the savor of long labor, and the younger the splendor of wilding nature. Both seek to become one with each and all.

"They cross the too-dry, sandy valleys made newly strange by the sin of vitacide, for which Eve and Adam fell, and to which their descendants remained blind.

"Re-forming family in the bright sun of continuing life, they bask in the vast plains of Missouria, scale rocky foothills, and shamble up the rough track to Cameron Pass.

"Crossing into a green-bottomed bowl with forested sides and rimy rim, they descend over deadfalls into darkness, over stream-slick rocks, rattlesnake holes, and crumbling ridges.

"They reach a time-stopped town, a last outpost of late modern ways, and camp in a deep field to dream of past delights and present adventure.

"Horse and bike at rest, uncle and niece walk toward a proud steeple that pierces the sky, arriving as church and courthouse disgorge the comforted, who go as one to continue conspicuous consumption, careless of earth, water, and sky.

"The pilgrims meet locals who conform and cannot form themselves, or offer hospitality, but a local family friend offers an evening picnic and hike into living beauty;

"And so the sojourners rest and meet their host next day after hours to drive west to a steep elk trail, and to walk up the Park Range.

"They pass stump-dotted scrub along a pined ridge as skinks scamper under glittering granite, raptors soar above, and resin and sage scent the cooling breeze;

"The earnest trio rise quickly as the dry air drinks their sweat and shady ravines of lodgepole pine, spruce and fir beckon. They tire, and seek out a lupine-carpeted ledge to refresh their flesh with water and flatbread, and their spirits with the valley vista.

"They mark the fitful drumming of flickers, the swaths of habitat that flourish and join all lives as one, and the deathly swathes that evince human error.

"As twilight falls, the host cannot find the way and panics, pulling the pilgrims into the darkness of horror at his inability to see, his failure to grasp control. Anxiety has mired him in the false safety of a dead past.

"The uncle recalls the way, the niece knows it and scrambles to a vantage point to show it, but the host protests mutiny and anarchy and will not follow.

"The pilgrims descend and hop a wagon to town; reporting the host's plight, they are taken into custody. The authorities prefer policing to progressing.

"The jailed uncle, a God-wrestler whose father spurned the law's spirit with its letter, ponders the laws as principles and speaks to the judge of a higher power and of co-creation, of character and responsibility, of the need for cure of gardens wild and tame.

"Deemed harmless, the pilgrims exit into the night. Drawn by light, they stop at a churchyard fête to buy sweet preserves and savory cheese and crusty bread for the journey;

"But the credit counter does not work, and the uncle fears to say that he can fix it as the helpless farmer calls for aid. The wary pilgrims leave their sustenance and retrieve their horse and bike to move north by moonlight in search of self-reliance and life-loving, life-sustaining change."

When Aaron finishes, the lights come up; he sees consternation on many faces, and disbelief in Rafa's. Feeling the cold clasp of remorse, he smiles wryly. The minister hops nimbly up on stage and rescues him, saying with evangelistic passion, "I thank our storyteller for sharing his juicy allegory, which bears witness to our earthly errors." She calls her flock to follow her to the hot pool, where they can sweat and cool off together and discern the pith of pilgrimage. They exit into the starry night, seemingly stunned by Aaron's bid for personal responsibility and self-policing as a cure for human error.

Soon only Rafa and Aaron remain, and she spits out a question through pursed lips: "Why did you lie? In Walden, you did what anyone with any sense would do, and they were vicious! They threw us in jail and called you The Jew and me The Darkey—they learned nothing from history! Why not reveal their evil?"

"I told a story to people who are no longer strangers to human error or its consequences, but who don't yet know what to do."

"A fairy tale?"

"A narrative they can use to pattern restoration," Aaron corrects.

"Shouldn't they have to pay penance?"

"They should reconcile with life in time, and they came a long way to do it."

Rafa shakes her head.

"You know how hard it is hard to make the change; we all do. The trick is to stop the influence of wrong changes, and failed ones."

Rafa shakes her head again.

"You've seen your family—your whole family—lose the way again and again. I wanted to inspire these pilgrims to touch the ground, to find a rock. They can find the way from there."

"A rock," she says pensively. After a smiling pause, she asks, "like Saint Peter?"

"And these stones," he says, pointing to her, and then to himself.

"I want to tell a real story, of what we saw outside Yellowstone. Will you help me?"

"Great choice! I'd be glad to."

"No poetry. Rhythm, maybe."

Over the next day, as Rafa struggles to write that story in the quiet of the sanctuary, Aaron sits with her to answer questions. A cloud of anxiety envelops him. He wonders if they have spent so much time together that the empathy that is coloring his care state is drawing her feelings toward him. He fills his core with strength, joy, and love of life, and shares them. When she taps her quill in frustration, and dips it in the ochre one too many times, he shifts to a cure state that is alert, expansive, off center, on edge. She moves forward, slightly frenzied, harnessing an old-time adrenal high, the fight or flight state used by aggressors and competitors. He wonders if it is coming from him, if some antigen or toxin is pushing his neurohumoral milieu into a subtle hell state. As Rafa writes away, he excuses himself and heads for the hot pool for a sweat ordeal to trigger relaxation.

By the time he returns to the rustic dining room in the old-style lodge of barked logs, she is gone; he is pleased to eat his dinner apart and in peace. This is all a bit much for him— and yet, when he arrives in the tea room that smells of sage and smoke and takes a seat by the glass-encircled hearth, he meditates easily on a fallen sugarpine branch from the foraging reserve. It is releasing its last traces of alluring resin as it warms the water in the glass brick walls secured with scattered metal screws. When Rafa takes her place by the mic and begins in a timid voice that soon swells with passion, his unease returns. He struggles to listen and to absorb her youthful wisdom.

She is telling the story of the day they left the Yellowstone Eden land and entered the Columbiana bioregion by way of the Jardine group, which stewards a recovering forest. Their school of habitat care emphasizes foraging, looking ahead to distant days when the descendants of moderns may know enough to go forth, multiply, and coevolve with life on earth. Aaron can see Jardine in his mind's eye: the cob houses spread out like giant toadstools that reminded him of romantic Swedish children's stories like *Snipp, Snapp & Snorum*, a book about little people that his grandmother translated as she read and he looked at the pictures. Aaron likewise recalls the old modern town of Gardiner that lies nearby, and that forms the center of a series of throwback strip malls and parking lots crammed with toxin-belching trucks and kindreds of insensitives.

Rafa perceived Jardine and Gardiner through the lens of her Sunday schooling, and transformed the story of their pleasant stay in one and their miserable passage through the other into a story of towns she calls Paul and Peter. Paul appears as a kindred that shares radiant, generous, inclusive love, and Peter as one of hard-headed rigidity. The former leads with faith, care, and love and the other with exclusion. Aaron's heart swells with pride. She has begun to forgive her father; she could not tell the tale this way if she had not. He can't believe now that he thought her homely at first, with a head of hair like one big cowlick, her face hunched inside round shoulders, and her eyes looking down or peering back—anywhere but at him. And now—perhaps because her posture has extended and pushed her face up like a flower—she is changing his very idea of beauty: expanding, refreshing, and inspiring it.

Suddenly, she stops. She has been speaking about the bloated homes of those residents of Gardiner who build new single family homes that hoard indoor space. A white-haired woman in front of her has delicately raised a hand. Aaron finds himself unaccountably angry at the interruption, just as he has been frightened and exhilarated by Rafa's storytelling. Rafa nods at the woman, who asks in a schoolmarmish tone, "Wouldn't you want to visit your grandma if she lived in such a fine home?"

Aaron feels vindicated when she replies, "I wouldn't need to be bribed to see a grandma—especially if she was a loving being who was—was ... "

Aaron suddenly feels like crying as Rafa's face flushes; she presses her lips together into a thin line, and drops her spunky, sassy sweetness to cry consternation into every open heart, "But my grandma was a doctor who got to care for others and not for me, and now she's died and I'll never get to meet her!"

Before he can think, Aaron is bounding somewhat ridiculously, off balance and on again, up to the stage. Standing beside Rafa, one arm on her shoulder, he says, "Whew! Now I know how a father feels. None of this is easy, and the loss of loved ones is especially hard, but we sure had a nice stay in that tiny little cramped loft in Jardine—I mean Paul—despite the indoor-outdoor toilet. We can safely say that our best hospitality—and this is saying something—has come from the Eden lands we have visited."

"*Tío*," Rafa says in a gentle tone of reproach.

The audience claps, and smiles parentally. Many have tears in their eyes. Rafa bows and steals away to the hot pool, where Aaron joins her; they sit side by side at the edge and dangle their feet in the water.

Aaron says, apologetically, "That sure was a good story."

Rafa laughs. "I think it needs a new ending."

Aaron laughs, "One without me in it."

"No, that was sweet."

Aaron sighs. He is not ready to be a father, yet cannot but conclude that he is developing the feelings of one. "I've been meaning to tell you, I checked the comm net, and there's still no tag out on you, no sign that anyone's searching for you. And, it looks like that group is offline. Someone may have … taken them out."

Rafa grunts in distress. "So it was all for nothing?"

"You're free, which is far from nothing, and you destroyed malicious devices, and you're going toward a new life that you can make your own. I'd say things came out well."

"I'm also in exile. I can't stop thinking of how Ma sent me away, like she wanted to get rid of me."

"I'm sure she did, but not for her sake, for yours."

Rafa sighs. After a time, she muses, "I've been thinking about missing the mark. About turning away from God and turning back, and I think I want to try and reconcile vitacide for my initiation and vocation projects."

"Big topic."

"Yes. And the question is not how did we get here, but what do we do now? How do we ascend from this low point on the rollercoaster ride of human cultural evolution?"

"Knowing your grandma, she's sent us on a mission that will have us solving some kind of problem that she didn't, and it will probably be a big one."

6

Portland

Wind-driven rain soaks Aaron, Rafa, Sleipnir, and their belongings, which are sitting on the dock at the Willamette River Terminal in Portland. The wind barge has gone on to its home dock, and the other passengers have scattered to go home or to find better shelter.

"Where's the downtown?" Rafa asks.

"We're in it. It looks like they turned the streets into a habitat! See the grid of fir trees?"

"No streets? You're right! It isn't like Denver. But how do they get around?"

He sees the flash of a bike and the bobbing of a jogger. "It looks like they have walker-biker trails, like these on the waterfront."

Rafa sees a line of cars skim a ridge and points to it. "And trams too. But the only buildings I see are along the river."

"I see glimpses of structures between the firs."

"Yes! And vertical gardens. And clearings over there."

"And mountains."

"And a river to the ocean! I've never seen an ocean."

"I haven't seen it since I was your age."

They hear dull steps on the dock and turn to see Doug, who is still big and spry but stooped. If not for the white bristles, and the scaly age spots that obscure his freckles, he would look seventy-six rather than ninety-six. He is approaching arm-in-arm with a woman whose radiance transfixes Aaron. She has sparkling amber eyes; full, bronze cheeks; a bright smile; long, dark hair; perfect posture and poise; as well as a voluptuous figure. When she reaches him, she extends her hand and says warmly, "I'm Parvati Kumar, the schoolteacher."

From somewhere in the hidden depths beneath his many years of celibacy comes a confusing surge of desire that impels him to offer an awkwardly anachronistic response. He takes her warm, slightly damp hand, and bows as he says, "And I am your faithful student."

Parvati laughs charmingly, and then says smoothly, "You'll have to come to the school and pattern that attitude for my youngest students."

Rafa's desire to please turns to dismay. Aaron's care state and Parvati's unfamiliar one coalesce like two clouds of invisible vapor that make one expansive state. One minute he was all Uncle, and now he is entranced by a bubbly beauty half his age. Rafa feels embarrassed—almost ashamed—of his confusion and of Parvati's role in it. She is relieved when Aaron turns to embrace Doug, and unprepared when Parvati throws her arms around Rafa's neck. Rafa returns the embrace and, feeling Parvati's state, does not want to let go. And so, in the very first encounter, Parvati changes both their lives.

"What is that? That state you're in?"

Parvati releases a peal of delighted laughter, draws back, and says, "It's a fertile state."

"It's exuberant, optimistic, delightful—and attracts care states," Rafa notes with a guttural chuckle.

Parvati blushes. "So that's what yours is!" she says, putting one arm around Rafa's shoulders so that both face Aaron and

Doug. "It's lovely—and so are you. I'm glad to see you so well recovered. The fertility students who come to us from Denver sometimes have to detox for a year before they can attune to the wild well enough to start our program."

"I hope—I hope my friend Mitzi is okay."

"We'll find out," Parvati says, with what seems to Rafa to be a perverse degree of confidence.

Doug says to Aaron, "I hear you need credits. Parvati can take you to a good dealer who'll give you a fair price for a horse with a history. And I hear that you, Rafa, need initiation and a vocation. I'm a trader, and you may as well take a look at that with me while we're here."

Parvati adds, "Yes, and first let's stow your things in the boat and take care of any errands you may have—like using the comm net."

"You haven't any on Saltspring?"

"There's one in town, but most of us are sensitives, and most of us use the biocomm."

"Without an interface?"

"That's right—we communicate directly over distance."

"Verbally?"

"More often in images or states, but some do chat."

"Where are the old glass and steel buildings?" Rafa asks.

"A lot were broken down and repurposed here and around Cascadia," Doug replies. "And a lot went to the Kilauea cauldron. Took a few loads myself on a schooner, but I don't pilot the big boats anymore."

"Where do people live?"

"Most live in hives—places where they live and work with a group. Most are modular pods made of local materials and stacked in an array, with permaculture on top. But each block and each neighborhood does things a bit differently."

"What if you can't walk or lift things?"

"Then you live on the river walk, or at a tram stop, or rely on a community. It's easier here than where you come from. People don't stay indoors much."

"Who's John?" Aaron asks hesitantly.

"An old friend of your mom, the doc who helped her work out the causes of her illness and started a clinic based on their ideas. You'll meet him in Saltspring. He was supposed to bring you out by train, but you got away from him."

"I wasn't ... fit for company ... until Rafa here came along."

"I wouldn't have known what to do without you," she says, not wanting to think of things having gone some other way.

"Well," says Parvati, "come with me, Aaron, and tell me all about your clinic in Amana, and what you learned there."

"And you can tell me what a legacy is."

"Sarah will talk to you about that. Let me catch you up on what we have and haven't done since you were last here." As they walk away, Parvati strokes Sleipner's neck and says, "We're leaving behind human exceptionalism, and destructive consumption, but we seem to be losing our esprit de corps, and our momentum ... "

"So, kid," Doug says to Rafa, pulling himself up to a lesser stoop and letting her pick up her gear, "how do you like Cascadia so far?"

"Things are not what they seem—they're better. There's light as well as dark."

Doug looks at her intently and asks about her education and experience. He seems to have a good idea of what she does not say, which saves her the wrench of telling all. Her avoidance may be short-sighted, but she is relieved to be free of her father's morbid attention to the dark, and also his mistrust of the light. Doug seems to notice that without prying. She likes him already, and he seems to see in her a kindred spirit; he says in a confidential tone, "I've got some trading to do while I'm here. If you help me, I can show you a few things."

Rafa knows enough to recognize a good offer. "Sure!"

Doug takes Rafa through the trader's Portland guild office and warehouse to the private marina where his forty-foot sloop is berthed. Rafa is amazed by the variety of boats: Doug points out a fleet of fishing boats, scattered river barges and taxis, and ocean-going wind vessels. Rafa hurries after him up the steps to his deck, waves as they pass his crew of five beautiful young women, and follows him into the hold to extricate a crate battened to a shelf. She maneuvers it awkwardly through the door and up the ladder to the deck, where she stops to let her arm muscles recover. She is amazed that a man as old and bent as Doug could be fit enough for trading.

She picks up the crate again, hoists it to her shoulder, and hurries to catch up with Doug, who is making his way along the maze of piers. Seeing his enthusiasm in action, Rafa smiles; it's contagious. She hopes that she too can go into trade.

Doug stops beside a huge schooner and hails its captain, Alex. Rafa sets the crate on the dock as a man descends from the foc's'le. He is short and barrel-chested, with curly gray hair and a full beard. Doug and Alex discuss a potential plan for moving ivory from Kodiak to Seattle, where a Duwamish artist will carve it to make inlay for a ceremonial Pan-Indian canoe paddle. The word ivory catches the attention of the crew from both this boat and others moored nearby. As the men talk, Rafa watches the crew unload the hold as if undoing a three-dimensional puzzle, and looks around at the astonishing variety of boat designs.

One catches her eye. It is an odd-looking saucer-shaped

fishing vessel that has a mast and rigging topped with a mesh ball. As Rafa watches, the ball whirrs and lines move forward through it. Aft of the ball, the lines are dotted with lures and hooks; forward of it, the lines are free of lures and hooks, and disappear over a metal crossbar and into a sleeve. Just as Rafa is wondering how a shallow vessel that has the shape of a coracle could make it through rough waters, its wind generator starts, lifting a gut spray skirt like that of a kayak and dropping a rudder as long as the mast.

Rafa hears Doug shout, "Rafa! Stop gawking and get down here!"

Doug's head disappears below the deck, and Rafa hoists the crate and bounds toward the ladder, catching up to him in the galley. Doug takes the crate and puts it on a fold-down table. He and Alex stand on opposite sides of it, both with arms folded, glaring at Rafa. She waits breathlessly for a reprimand—but the older men burst into laughter.

"We're just playing roles," Doug says. He gestures to Alex and says, "This is my long-time part-time partner in trade, Alex. He's a gnome. I mean he's from Nome. Alex, this is Rafa, the granddaughter of one of my best and oldest friends." The captain smiles broadly, reaches for Rafa's hand, and pumps it like a human-powered generator. "Good to meet you! Any friend of Doug's is a friend of mine. My boat is your boat—to crew on or to trade with!"

"Everything's in the walls," Rafa observes, looking at the floor-to-ceiling storage hooks, shelves, and compartments.

"It's like the interior of my Nome home," Alex says proudly. "My wife is crazy about her Japanese and T'lingit roots. She designs tatami longhouses. We used that here," he says, pointing to the wall above the table. "The table folds up over all of this."

Rafa sees a round-cornered rectangular groove corresponding to the shape of the table. Inside the groove are a fold-down box light, an altar inset with tea lights and incense burners, a tiny wet bar, and a light box with a brightly backlit photo of a massive mountain. Rafa scans the room and realizes that every square centimeter of the interior is a hatch that doubles as furniture.

Alex points to the photo. "That's Denali, prime destination of peak pilgrims. The light is for phototherapy. I can't winter over without it."

"Winter over?"

"Adapt to the winter darkness of the far north. I grew up there, but never adapted. The Inuits on the crew can do it, but they'd rather go to Hawaii."

Rafa is amazed. She had studied the Arctic in school, but thought of it the way she thought of Ancient Greece, as a collection of myths and tall tales.

"Okay," Doug says, holding out two pocket liquor flasks while Alex retrieves a large bamboo box from a low cabinet. "Let's cut to the chase. Your job—Rafa—is to find all of the metal pellets in the venison bags—and I mean every single tiny fragment of metal—and put them in these flasks. Put the venison in this box. Alex and I are going to the market. When we return, you and I have to get ourselves back up and over to a client's office before meeting Parvati and Aaron for lunch. You'll have to stay focused."

"Why the flasks?"

"I use them for private cargo that's worth enough to draw malefactors."

"Doug will have enough to pay his bills and to retire—and to pay for Sarah's retirement, if she's willing to leave her nest."

"If Aaron succeeds, she may join me," Doug says.

"Use this bowl," Alex says to Rafa, retrieving a pressed metal plate with a high rim from a cabinet. "Empty a bag in here and hunt and peck the pellets."

"Hunt and peck?"

Alex laughs. "Like a chicken feeding. Where have you been all your life?"

"In a city."

"Sorry to hear it," Alex says.

Rafa smiles. The men ascend the ladder, talking of the venison market in Missouria. Rafa takes a few minutes to set up a system. She puts the crate on the floor and puts a few bags on the table beside the bowl and flasks. Soon she is opening a cellophane bag, pouring its contents into the bowl, transferring pellets to the flasks, and returning venison to a bag that she tosses in the box. She works steadily and consistently, her focus so intent that she is aware of nothing else until she screws the lids on the flasks, pockets them, and returns the cellophane bags to the crate.

She sits down to rest and reflect on trade, and the strength and stamina and wide array of skills that it entails. Just as she is becoming impatient, she hears Doug call, "Time to go!"

"Do you want to check my work?"

"Hand up the box," Doug replies curtly, "and the booze."

Rafa follows instructions. She wonders how much of Doug's talk is misdirection. The answer comes to her as she heaves the crate above her shoulders: everything Doug says is misdirection wrapped around a hidden purpose that she can't see. Soon Doug and Rafa have said goodbye to Alex and are walking under a long awning by the river and into the marketplace that dominates the riverfront near the trader's marina. The marketplace is made up of pods stacked in a complex pattern and joined by stairs and walkways. Most pods open to a central courtyard. As Rafa admires the astonishing array of fresh produce, handcrafted furniture, woven blankets, and painted clothing that they pass, Doug shares stories and pearls that open a view into the traders' guild.

"Information is currency you get by staying alert. Be generous and trade openly, but not one-sidedly—or blindly. And fill in any blanks accurately. People can't tell you what they don't know and won't tell you what they don't want to. Many of them fail to grasp the obvious truth that for cost-based currencies to flow sustainably, ideas and information have to flow freely."

Doug goes on in that vein, and Rafa absorbs it all as best she can. Later, when they have passed many vendors, they reach his client's enclosure. Doug presses the flesh, weighs the flasks, and trades news. After a while, he and his client, a wizened Inuit woman of Doug's generation, begin to reminisce with Rafa as their audience.

"The most money we ever made together was on a dozen young yaks," Doug says. "I picked them up in Hawaii and brought them here in the '30s. I was just learning to sail solo. I had one passenger—the agro guilder who kept the yaks and planned to go on with them to Hudson Bay."

"I remember!" she says with a wide smile. "They were priceless—already extinct in the wild. The modern traders who didn't know how to harvest their wool had been skinning them and trading the skins."

"I was shit scared. I couldn't hide them. I couldn't get a warrior. I had to count on not meeting anyone who might guess their worth, and on my agro guilder being one of the two people alive who knew how to raise them."

"No cash value to anyone else," she nods sagely. "Best strategy."

"Like the seal blubber you sold me on our first trade. The fertility school had grown too fast and the kitchen at the center was out of calories. You told me how Arctic people sacrificed their own seals and could find no outside market for the blubber. So you got me some flash-frozen blubber."

"I wanted to show you our young singles, but you said no. Perhaps your young friend here would like to buy a mate."

Rafa cannot conceal her shock. When she recovers, she says, "No, thank you."

Doug and his fellow trader burst into laughter. Doug says, "Gotcha!"

The old woman says to Doug, "I remember when you carried warriors."

Doug shakes his head. "Before they had a fleet, I took them wherever they needed to go. Malefactors assumed I was carrying precious cargo. Most of the malefactors were former mercenaries. They go feral fast, but they don't think like traders—lucky for us. They trained our warriors by attacking my boats—over and over again."

"That's when you lost the yawl."

The friends go on reminiscing. After a time, Doug leads Rafa out of the market and back to the marina, where he says, "You can tell your uncle that when the old currencies collapsed and the circuses in Ottawa and Washington fell apart, Cascadia's new economy was already in full flow."

"When was that?"

"No particular time. That's old age talking. It wasn't a collapse—it was a decline. Those years were great for mockers like me. Failure fuels satire."

"Do you trade in silver?" Rafa asks to avoid mentioning the pellets she put in his flasks.

"It's okay. I carry a very sensitive device detector—my old brain. I can pick up listening devices better than most communicators." Doug looks around. "We can talk. The pellets were titanium. A fabro designer on Van Island makes submersibles for deep-water repairs at the new tide generator in Victoria. I trade in salvaged metal only—even though it costs me to verify it and keeps me sharp trading it. Reduces toxic waste."

"That shipment must have been worth millions of credits! Shouldn't you have brought a warrior?"

"The metal is worth what the client will pay, which is a lot because my client can trust me to get high quality salvage. My trustworthiness is my most important protection. I wear it on my sleeve, and I do everything I can to make it very, very expensive to steal from me. You'd have to follow me and know everything I know and predict my behavior. That would take a full-time tail, and even malefactors have to cover their costs—and control their people."

"Is that how you earn credits?"

"First, I usually trade in goods and favors that most people value a little, like the liquor I bring to local watering holes. That keeps us all in business, which means that traders and locals who like to drink—which is almost all of them—have my back at all times. Two, I charge prices clients and customers want to pay—cost plus sustainability. I take a living wage and pay the same to my crew, and profit every now and then with windfalls like this. Three, I trade in cargoes like venison that have no resale value. Only Sarah and a few others will buy it, because most clients who eat it raise their own deer to be sure it's safe. Four, if a client orders something costly, I'll say I'll try to get it and don't know if or when I can, and then bring it when they least expect it."

"So … a trader should be predictable as far as integrity and reliability but otherwise unpredictable."

"Hmmm. Not necessarily. Most people are unpredictable

because they don't know what they're doing or can't get up to speed. Incompetence has its upside—but it costs money and drives up prices. Clients don't like that. The trader ends up lying or stealing or folding."

"So I should be honest and wily and competent and what? What else?"

"Good question. The best traders, and I'm one of them, improvise. We figure things out in the moment, trade by trade. I learned that from John's music. I track costs of trade chains and goods and trade in the moment to suit the time and place and client. And I respond to offers by the end of the business day at the latest. Clients like a quick turn-around. No one likes uncertainty."

"That isn't one thing, that's a lot of things!"

"Exactly. It's a way of life that develops over time—an art like any other."

"So you're telling me to be experienced."

Doug laughs. "I'm telling you to get experience and use it wisely."

"Oh, that's all," Rafa says ironically.

"And to use the hard-won wisdom of others—me for starters."

7

Salish Sea

Three days later, they have finished their business in Portland; headed north over the Pacific—which made Rafa too seasick to thrill to the scenery; gone up the strait between the Olympic Peninsula and Van Island; and finally headed north on the Salish Sea along the mainland coast. Today, the sky is leaden and the wind blows steadily from the south-southeast. Doug's boat cuts smoothly through the low chop on autopilot, its sails taut and its mast heeled thirty degrees. Aaron, Rafa, and Parvati are sitting with Doug on the bench behind the helm.

"I can't believe how much Seattle has changed—and Bellingham," Aaron says. "We drove through them on our first visit. I know it's been a long time, but I expected to see some of the tall buildings—in Seattle especially, given the urbanization policy of thirty-five years ago. Where did all that metal go?"

"Some of it went into the cauldrons at Etna after the big quake," Parvati replies. "Alan died in that quake, you know. He came visiting at the wrong time. And Doug was nearly caught in the tsunami that came before it. You can still see the scars on the ocean shores. Anyway, my family, who are also traders, took some of the salvage from both disasters to Australia to build pods, and to China to frame homes against future quakes."

"What about the glass?" Rafa asks.

"I think most of it was repurposed."

"Is that what you wanted us to see?" Aaron asks Doug.

"I'm just taking you up the coast so you can see the forest."

"The forest? The woods are pretty patchy. Would you call them forest?"

"I'd call them forest in some of the bottom lands."

"We've seen healthy arable and pasture."

"In the bottom lands. Did you notice the naked peaks? And the steep slopes that haven't recovered from the Forest Service's repeated clear cuts of up to thirty years ago—the ones that recovered badly and then burned?"

"I noticed blanks in the high places. I thought maybe that's where the glaciers were."

"Good call. They're gone from heat. That and intentional and careless destruction and the resulting climate instability played a part in the stripping of the mountains."

"On the way out, we saw a lot of areas that were spared, especially in Mississippia, where the arctic fronts still come down."

"It's worse out here—just the reverse of what we expected when we all moved out here to be near the lush forests of Cascadia. And this," Doug declares triumphantly, "is what I want you to see."

"What?" Rafa asks.

"Look at the land and tell me what you notice about the habitat here."

"Well, it looks like some crazy giant made a huge gash along the earth and mowed one side of it."

"Good. Aaron?"

"I don't want to know what it is. But I do. It's the old border, isn't it?"

"Right. Two giants made that gash."

"Why is the old Canada so much healthier?"

"You probably weren't paying attention to Canada back in 2029. I trace it to the big quake. The government started paying loggers and others who earned their living by destroying crown lands to restore them instead. They even created some irrigated reserves and areas where the land belonged to itself. Some are Eden lands now—they can thrive without human labor. Some say they're the reason the oxygen level is as high as it is today—that and the policies that saved the Finnmark and Patagonia."

"I thought it was healthy," Rafa says sadly. "I didn't see it right."

Rafa has the sudden sense that the closed cylinder in which she had been living has expanded in all directions. This is her first embodied realization of humanity's encroachment on life. She is feeling what is happening to the body of life as if it were happening to her. It reminds her of the feeling of awakening in one of the berths below and being aware of the others on the boat generating a kind of grid of radiant life energy. It is dizzying—almost overwhelming—and also exhilarating. It is changing her relation to life in space and time.

"Why hasn't the alpine forest recovered?" Rafa asks.

Doug replies, "Some say it was the fall in oxygen, but I think that was a consequence. Others blame rising temperatures, or decreasing rainfall, or changes in ocean currents."

Aaron says, "Analysis doesn't help. You can't point to any one factor. You could say that consumptive destruction caused all of it."

"What about the theory that there was a change below the earth's crust, in the molten core and magnetosphere?" Parvati asks.

Aaron smiles slyly. "Maybe that's what made us cut down the forests. Or maybe it was the old toxic comm system."

"Let's face it," Doug says. "We all know what did it: us. Humans. And we don't know what to do about it."

"Sarah's been doing more than her share—and my family did too. Mom taught me to get a feel for clusters of problems and for sets of actionable solutions—and for ways to bridge them," Aaron says sanguinely.

"You mean, work forward from problems and backward from solutions?" Rafa asks.

"Exactly. And do it on the human and habitat scales at the same time. Civilizations as we knew them—the gathering in cities, breaking ties to habitats, decimating interbeing—had to stop for good. Our species kept falling from Eden as from Eridhu. Time to retire that mistake."

Doug says, "Well, you didn't see the old pattern in Portland and you won't find it in Van city."

"What is Vancouver like now?" Aaron asks.

Parvati says, "Van's thriving. People loved it too much to leave it. When it lost the old consumptive-destructive trade, and Vic got out in front with its emerging trader's hub, Van developed its old centers for learning and the arts. They bill the old university as a discovery center. The faculty trains fine artists and artisans, and performing artists for all media. At the graduate level, they train knowledge developers and keepers for contemplative subjects like pure math, philosophy, theology, and astrophysics. They even support the development of New Renascence vocations."

"I'd like to know more about that," Rafa says.

Doug says, "I know you would. That's why we're going to Van. You'll see something of the old U of C," Doug says to Aaron. "Boundary crossers in majors like the old Ideas and Methods. Committees like Social Thought and Virology."

Aaron muses, "It isn't so long since ideas were valued apart from their monetary value."

"It sure feels long," Doug says with a dark laugh. "But Van has really taken the baton. The whole city is a living laboratory for large-scale ventures in experimental systems for things like transportation and eco-villages and habitat commons."

"It has a reputation for comm development. The film bank supports a huge online archive that includes all kinds of media," Aaron says.

Parvati says, "I know them from their medical archive. If you want an image of Damien or Maimonides or Vesalius or Osler, you can find it in their archive in seconds."

"Why medical?"

"I wrote your legacy transmission."

"I see. Actually I don't."

"You will," she says with a sly smile. Returning to the topic, Parvati adds, "And the archive doesn't enable addictions to virtual reality or devices. If you're on too often or too long, they suspend you."

"They're a bit too quick for me. I'm not as fast as I used to be! And so the ageism of the old Internet lives on," Doug says.

They fall quiet after that, and Aaron finds himself brooding; when he notices it, he also feels Doug's eyes on him. He has tried to appear cheerful, and to deflect suspicion by talking of mourning his mother, but he guesses that Doug has seen through his ruses, and is unsurprised when Doug says, "You don't seem too keen on this circuit."

Aaron feels chilled. He can no longer tell if it's the wind over the water, the tedium of cruising, or some kind of deterioration in his flesh. Aaron struggles to orient his body to this moment in this place. He watches the shore go by in hopes of grounding his mind in matter. He wants to be open, but doesn't want to compromise the time that remains, and he knows that Doug's life expectancy is short, and that his own may be even shorter.

Aaron finally says, "Lots to think about."

Doug nods. "Let me know if you want to talk about it."

"Thanks. I will."

Later, Aaron and Rafa stand in front of a yellow cedar sculpture entitled, "The Raven and the First Men." A plaque says that it was carved by a man named Bill Reid, and that it was placed at this site seventy years ago. It was part of the Museum of Anthropology of the University of British Columbia, which is now the Museum of Origins and Endings of the city-wide Discovery Nexus. The sculpture was carved from a massive block of wood made from the trunks of several venerable trees, and depicts a local creation story in which a large raven is opening a shell out of which climb the first humans. When Aaron was young, he saw it as challenging modern ideas of mechanism; now it seems to him to invite haunting questions about human endings, allegorical and material.

Aaron talks easily to Rafa about the origins and endings defined by astronomical, geological, biological, and evolutionary time scales; about the timelines defined by habitats and species; about rites of passage in the human lifecycle; and about how each source of life adds to the dynamic body of life in time. Rafa's mind is like a garden that has been richly seeded and needs thinning; she has taken in so many ideas that they have become dense and tangled and are blocking out the light. The most intensive gardener is Parvati, who has given Rafa a short history of Cascadia and its falling birth rates, the unexpected rapidity of the New Exodus from areas of urban sprawl, and the revival of creative, artisanal local living economies.

Diversity of production is one of Doug's favorite topics, being as it is the greatest impetus behind trade. Rafa feels tenderly toward him, as to a grandfather who is brave as he nears the end of his days. She begins to take a different view of origins. She considers the course of her life—how she will join the origin and end—and begins to see her vocation as a route through time and place. She clears a space in her body for a germ of the future. The emptiness is daunting. She has never considered what it might be like to be pregnant with the future, or to create something lasting. She is unnerved by the realization that the coming change will not be another pilgrimage; she must remain committed and allow her course to grow into the future like a branch of the tree of life that is always seeking the sun.

They soon reach the exhibition ground west of the museum, where they stop at a cart to taste perennial foods of the region: grilled chanterelles, colorful dried berries and smoked salmon. They wander through an exhibit of the major watersheds of the world and cultures to which they gave birth. When they go out to wait at a tram stop by the horticulture garden, a lone player serenades them with a Scottish bagpipe. Soon, they board a solar tram to Stanley Park and disembark in the weak light of late afternoon opposite a field packed with colorful, flag-topped tents.

"Were these here this morning?" Rafa asks in confusion.

"No," Aaron says. "What's going on?"

"This is the Artisans' School," Doug replies.

"It's a traveling school," Parvati explains as they cross the tram line and approach the nearest row of tents. "They come every season. This time of year they teach harvest crafts—food preservation, grass and reed weaving, hardtack baking, and gourd decoration and carving."

"They sell their own, too," Doug says. "It's a great way to start a business."

Parvati says enthusiastically, "I love the fall session! It's usually the biggest one. They probably invited the regular teachers—the ones who hold classes in pottery, weaving, dying, spinning, decorative painting—and artists and performers, too. We may see some spectacles tonight."

"Its like a traveling circus—but participatory," Aaron says.

Parvati laughs. "It is—and it isn't. There's nothing else like it."

Aaron says, "Where did the tents and supplies come from?"

Doug says, "Their boats probably anchored near mine. And they're probably selling food from their last location, which means we can forage right here."

Rafa says, "Let's eat! That snack was like a teaser."

"After I buy a hat," Doug interjects, "for anyone who wants one."

Rafa is surprised at Doug's energy as he enters the foyer of a large, felted-wool tent dyed in pink and purple and tries on some of the hats that are hanging from a fishnet suspended under the tent top. As he tries one after the other—a vintage green fedora, a classic black top hat, a red bark bowler hat, a bearskin hat, and a kufi with a geometric pattern—he finally picks a plaid ascot cap and asks Rafa, "What do you think?"

She puts on a vintage sun hat and tips her head to consider his new look. "Perfect! And practical. What do you think of mine?"

"You look lovely, but a bit prim. I see you in a tuque."

"Do you think so?"

The proprietor is like a man whose home has been invaded by a rowdy crowd of strangers. He asks politely, but with a touch of anxiety, "Can I help you?"

"Yes, a hat for each of us, and an inside tip on the best food cart."

Fifteen minutes later, after Doug has spent too many credits on hats, scarves, and gloves and Rafa is feeling cozy, they go to a row of food carts near the center row of tents and choose street foods to suit their tastes. After, they feel warm and satisfied and sanguine as they set off on the boardwalk to visit the Film Bank, which Doug tells them is several miles away and will be open around the clock. So, they have no appointments and no need to hurry. As the sun approaches the horizon, Doug stops and rests his arms on the sea wall railing to look across Burrard Inlet and watch mist gather over North Van and Grouse Mountain.

Rafa asks, "Do you think I should learn a craft while we're here?"

Doug replies, "No. You'd be better off learning from Björn, or at the Nexus. The fall fair is for children and hobbyists and people integrated into remote habitats, not for guilders."

"Look!" Parvati exclaims excitedly. She disappears up the boardwalk.

"What is it?" Rafa asks.

"I don't know, but I think we'll find out when we catch up to her."

They walk slowly, enjoying the last daylight views of the waterfront and keeping the pace set by the oldest members of their little party. Soon Aaron notices a group of performers on the west wall of an old twelve-story modern building on the other side of a paved plaza.

Rafa asks, "What are they doing?"

Aaron asks, "Is that safe?"

"Probably not," replies Doug.

They watch as several abseilers move back and forth over the wall, weaving their ropes into a giant lanyard as they descend. In the declining daylight, the ropes are both lit by natural light and backlit by the building's interior lights. Parvati points out that they—or they and other teams—have been covering the wall with vertical weavings in a wide variety of colors and patterns. Aaron stands with her, side-by-side, enjoying the revelation of the installation, which strikes him as unaccountably romantic. "I could stand here all night."

They are startled when a string band starts up, and follow the sound to the center of the plaza, where musicians are gathering on ledges and paving stones.

"Look!" Parvati says. "The abseilers are keeping time."

"When you're done looking at that, come look at the pavement beyond them. The chalk artists have roped off an area and sketched the works they'll be completing over the next few days," says Doug.

The group spends the next half hour enjoying the music, the art, and the dancing abseilers. Doug rests on a bench and stays there through a series of French Canadian and Irish fiddle tunes, after which the group continues along the boardwalk, which is now illuminated by borders dotted with strips of tiny solar lights.

"What are they doing?" asks Aaron. "The boats on the Inlet?"

Doug leans over the sea wall railing. "It's a water festival!"

"Are they—are those boats following the patterns set by the abseilers?"

Doug watches them and says, "No. But they are tracing patterns—something you can do with boats powered by solar-wind turbines. It's fun—and takes a lot of concentration."

"Looks like synchronized swimming," says Rafa.

"Let's look through a telescope," Parvati says, leading the group to one of the telescopes that stand at intervals along the sea wall. Once their turn comes around, Parvati looks through and, after a gasp, says, "They're doing some kind of diving! What is it?"

Doug stands on the circular step at the base of the telescope and eyes the boats. "If a crew member makes a mistake they have to walk the plank—which is one way of getting ready for the New Year polar bear swims."

Aaron decides to make a holiday of their last night here. "I'm going to give the Film Bank a miss. The last thing I need is another visit to an archive."

"Why don't we go back to Doug's boat and sail out toward those boats," asks Rafa. "That would be so much fun!"

"In a minute." Doug inhales deeply. "This is my favorite view in the world—and my favorite city. Vancouverites kick-started the new economy—they were out ahead of Barcelona and Buenos Aires and Kuala Lumpur. They set the bar high and have led ever since—and still know how to have a good time."

8

Research Station

T he first thing that strikes Sarah on seeing Aaron and Rafa
is the way that they stare all around in wonderment—or
perhaps confusion—as they walk toward her along the road
to the lodge. First, she sees them point to the linear foraging
garden that forms a colorful understory along the roads and
paths, and is now featuring fall chanterelles and salmon berries.
Then they stop to admire and discuss the sod-roofed group
houses made of cob; the small pasture with sheds, ponds, and
mounds for compost and soil production; the agricultural—or
agro—center with its barn, dairy, and seaweed feeders for sheep,
goats, ducks, and chickens; and the large pasture between the
agro center and the lodge. There they stop again, noticing some
of the centers nestled in the forest around the lodge: the school
on the left beyond the pasture; the fertility center with visiting
student housing; the forest theater with its living alder tree oval
and water features; the hot houses and outdoor gardens; and the
forest sanctuary near the steep slopes that fall away south to the
valley, where their orchards and apiaries line the road to Fulford.

Sarah's heart swells with grandparental love and a touch of
vanity as she smiles at her beloved visitors who are like rubes
from the past—he from nineteenth century Iowa and she from
the Denver backwater that is set to move toward oblivion. Sarah
was the first of her friends and family to leave her pointless

bureaucratic management job; to join in the New Exodus by moving to the old trailer behind her sister's farm; and then to this New Monastic community, one of the first to engage in a continuing experiment in restoration and renewal. She can't wait to share it with Aaron, whose mother was—in retrospect—more responsible for the formation of this community than anyone else.

Sarah has, perhaps, stayed alive for Aaron's visit to this community, which seems to her to be losing its bloom. Since the deaths of the founders, she has been the keeper of its story, its primary historian, narrator, and guide, like the stage manager character in the Thornton Wilder play *Our Town* who can hear the living and dead. She has stepped into the role of visionary and futurist, which has made her aware of her limitations as its leader and governor and spirit-keeper, and of the fact that something has been missing since Melissa decided not to join her old friends here. They have had astonishing success in reframing human fertility as restoring and enhancing the body of life, but their work has become unbalanced: they do too little for the body of humanity as it manifests here, in this place. They are not refreshing themselves well enough to remain a wellspring for the renewal of evolved life.

As Aaron spots her waiting in front of the main entrance, and waves to her, she can see that anxiety clouds his bright smile. Rafa, who never knew her grandmother Melissa, is looking at Sarah warily, and hanging back while Aaron steps forward to embrace her. Their heartache joins and swells. Both release tears as Sarah says, "I'm so sorry for your loss."

Rafa's eyes widen and she looks away, perhaps upset to see her uncle cry. Releasing Aaron, Sarah sweeps Rafa into a loving hug that Rafa receives stiffly until she melts into Sarah's warm hug. "Welcome, granddaughter of my dearest friend. Please feel free to consider me as another grandmother whenever you like."

"You have that same state as Parvati, but stronger, bigger," Rafa says.

Sarah draws back and examines Rafa. "Speaking of Parvati, and her fertile state, where is she?"

"She went into the park to gather berries for Cookie."

"Ah, of course; he can't get enough of those. And Doug?"

"He's bringing the cart up from the dock."

Sarah nods. "Of course. You know you are the incarnation of your grandfather—but your cheekbones are higher and broader, like Melissa's. And your eyes are darker … "

"Dad says I look like an Ashkenaz, like him," Rafa says. "But Mom says I look like a Mayan."

"They marry happily in you. Come, now, give me your crowns."

Sarah reaches out her hands, and Aaron feels her warm palm on his scalp. When she is done muttering a blessing under her breath, she lifts her palms and asks, "Is Doug bringing tropical fruits?"

"Yes!" Aaron replies.

"Good. We plan to grow those in the new tropical hot house. I saw you looking at the grounds; we'll tour them later. For now, I'd like to take you in for a get-acquainted tea"

"Doug and Parvati were very mysterious about the legacy."

"What did they tell you?"

"Only that you would have to explain it, and that Parvati prepared enactments of my mother's life and the Center's beginnings."

"She seems to know more about *Tío* than he does," Rafa interjects.

"She was always curious about and drawn to the story of your family. I think she got to feeling close to you as she interviewed me and Doug and John." Seeing Aaron frown at her mention of John, Sarah adds, "Come in and see the lodge on our way to morning tea. I'll explain more when we're settled."

Aaron follows Sarah and Rafa up the stairs and through the wide entry door, which is solid wood carved with images of salmon. As they pass through it, Sarah describes salmon as the fertilizer of the forest, spread by the bears who fish for them in the streams. In the entry foyer, they take off their shoes, leaving them in the cubbyholes on either side. Aaron pauses to admire the bright, diffuse light that is focused by a roof lens, then transmitted and magnified through reflecting tubes that illuminate the art glass fixtures of the ceiling. The latter serve as light spreaders and down lights. The trio continue through a long, quiet hall with a soft runner that Aaron recognizes as a rya rug like the ones his mother made. He notices the sconces that hold oil lamps during rites and festivals, and realizes that he is already familiar with the lodge from times when he called Sarah for his mother and stayed on the call long enough to see and hear her news.

When they exit the hall into the common room, Aaron stops in amazement; memory carries him back to his last visit, forty years ago. The room has changed very little. The glass-paned doors on the right reveal that the dining room beyond is also much the same. Both great rooms are paneled with warm, lacquered cedar that was cut and polished when the land was cleared, and they share a monumental fireplace—now retrofitted to burn beeswax candles—fashioned with local river stones. He can see the old, sturdy dining tables and chairs in the other room, and in the common room the familiar grouping of wooden armchairs and settees softened and brightened by colorful cushions and a thick hearthrug. Beyond the hearth stand tables with wooden chairs, groupings of armchairs, and—in a far corner—a low stage with musical instruments. Standing against the walls are new cabinets and shelves filled with books, games, puzzles, and art materials, some of them modern antiques and some made on site.

Now, the rooms are—like the foyer—flooded with natural light that reveals the walls to be decorated with tapestries designed and woven by fabro guilders seeking membership in the fiber sub-guild. Aaron notes that all of the new elements are contextual, so that the evolving décor offers pleasing variety and contrast and yet also advances a single vision. Aaron is still staring at the walls when Sarah gently takes his arm and leads him into a private dining room on the left, closing the glass-paneled door after them. The room's sideboard is set for tea and cookies, and its windows overlook the garden to the north and the trail to the forest sanctuary to the east. On the far wall is an exit that leads to a small porch which in turn leads to a network of mulched trails.

Sarah pours the hot water into the pot on the tea tray; places cream, sugar, and a plate of cookies on the tray; and carries it to a long narrow dining table set at a diagonal. Above it is a central light spreader, and on it a fine monk's path tablecloth. As Aaron and Rafa take seats that look out to the forest east of the lodge and to the rocky summit beyond the garden to the north, Sarah sits and waits for the tea to brew. She tells them that this dining room has been reserved for Aaron through the end of the enactments that transmit his legacy, and that the reservation may be shortened or lengthened according to his wishes.

As she pours out the tea, Aaron sees Sarah and Doug in his mind's eye, remembering them from childhood and also as they are now. Doug was a head taller then, broad-shouldered and agile, with thick brown hair, freckled cheeks, and a sturdy nose reddened by the sun. He had favored a smart-aleck grin, and his goading signaled disrespect for Sarah and the whole wide world. Her beautiful narrow features, pale skin, and long blond hair formed a perfect frame for her flashy smile, and her placid disregard for Doug's antics—along with her large-breasted earthiness—made her seem both anchor and foil for Doug's eternal childhood.

They had stayed at the family home in Denver then, but never at the same time. Sarah stayed for weeks while training as a yoga teacher, and wore a thick French braid and clothes that showed off her posture and fitness. Doug would drop in without warning and stay only long enough to confide in Melissa and get her advice. He was a moody businessman then, mythically successful in Silicon Valley but happiest in leathers and in his role as a big, no-nonsense biker. Sarah is taller than Doug now, but her long white hair is still fixed in the usual braid, and her posture remains in fine form, as do the facial bones that sustain her features. Her billowy white robes nearly conceal the loose flesh that hangs from her upper arms. Doug, in contrast, is bent; his nose aims toward his chin like the beak of a hawk, and his attitude seems set against submersion in this rich sea of forest air.

Neither had a child, Aaron thinks wistfully, *so they borrowed me*. His heart is divided between the love that rises to meet theirs and the sorrow he feels in the thought that they will soon follow his mother into earth and ether.

Once the tea has been poured and Sarah has had a sip of it and a bite of shortbread, Aaron says, "Mom was mysterious at the last. She spent her last hours with John, who I didn't recognize, and then she made me promise to come here. She didn't explain a thing. I felt like she'd left me with a double mystery."

Sarah reaches out to put her hand on his upper arm and asks,

"Can you be strong?"

Anxiety creeps up Aaron's back. "I like to think so."

"The legacy is a process of creative transformation that takes as much or more time that earning initiation or vocation."

"Why did she tell me about it at the last minute?"

Sarah locks Aaron's gaze and continues sweetly, "It took a long time for her to see that you belonged here, now, with us."

"How could I belong here?"

Sarah says gently and slowly, watching his expression carefully, "As you may know, the future of life in time remains uncertain."

Rafa's brows shoot upward under her fringe of hair. No one she knows has ever spoken forthrightly about what Aaron contradicts in dismay. "No! The body of life is recovering! Everywhere Rafa or I went, we encountered cities and communities practicing Carson purification and Suzuki restoration—or better. Last year, the Rift Valley Field University measured four inches of snow on Mount Kilimanjaro! And temperatures in hot zones have been falling for ten years running!"

Sarah replies gently, "Unfortunately, the Great Poisoning continues to spread, to undo our habitat restoration and to imperil the future of life. We don't know if humanity will outlive the radical and reckless experiments of the modern era. And our own center is growing weaker just when it needs to grow stronger."

"I'm very sorry to hear that, but what does that have to do with me?"

"Do you want a minute before we go on? We could finish our tea, and let the fragility of our work as a species sink in before we look ahead."

Aaron nods. They drink tea in silence. Aaron's breathing

becomes rapid and then slows. Sarah can feel his tension, and notices that Rafa is not surprised or distressed. The possibility that humans will vanish from Earth is not new to her. Sarah relaxes, and soon Aaron breathes more easily.

"Perhaps you could tell us about the legacy now?"

"Yes, perfect." Sarah leans back, looking up at the light spreader as she collects her thoughts. "Our ways have evolved rapidly. That was one of the reasons that your mother was wary of us and never came to visit. She liked to try new things slowly for fear of unforeseen consequences, and because her illness made her cautious. I didn't like to press her to visit, both for those reasons and because she had already done enough. I didn't even tell her when we changed our name to the Saltspring Island Research Station. That was when the Friday Harbor Station closed and its scientists moved here, and told us we were different than most of the experimental communities because we are strong in rational and scientific thinking."

"Is that why you wanted her to make the journey? To share medical science?"

"Naturally. I've come to think that we're losing steam because our work is incomplete. We never cared for the sick. We have no doctor. We don't practice care or cure of ailments. The root of our philosophy split in two: one shoot is fertility and fertile restoration of the body of life, and the other is human restoration through medicine—the kind that your mother and John developed. I wanted your mom to come to stay with us and figure out how to mend the split."

"But what's Aaron's legacy?" Rafa asks urgently.

"We view life as comprising three phases. The first is preparation, which culminates in initiation and vocation."

"We have that in Denver," Rafa says.

"And you can finish here. The second phase is lifework, which extends from around twenty to sixty years of age. That's where we become useful to the body of life and restore it through our work—or support those who do. The last phase, which is a bit like the forest years in Hinduism, is the legacy."

"You mean it's like elderhood?"

"It's analogous, but those of us who choose to do a legacy project bring our life experiences to fruition, and then use them to change the future."

"So, it's the work we leave behind us?"

"It's the immortality of the meaning and purpose that we have co-created in our lives, and that we transform to complete a gift to our descendents to use in forming a living future."

"For example?"

"For example, the founders created this community, and your mother and John their clinics."

"And I would do what?" Aaron can no longer hold back hot tears; mourning and despair mingle. "We gave up everything. I'm worn out. And I haven't finished mourning Mom's death."

"You need respite, and you'll have it. Find someone to replace you in the Amanas, mourn your mother, take whatever time you need to get to know us, and then receive your legacy transmission. After that, take whatever more time you need to decide whether to accept it."

"What if he doesn't want to do that for you?" Rafa asks protectively, taking his hand.

"The legacy doesn't work that way. The transmission is for telling the part of Aaron's life story that preceded his first visit here, so that he can—with all of us—can revisit his formation from the point of view of a fully mature and experienced adult. The next phase is a ritual followed by several months of contemplation, during which Aaron can consider his life and discern what he intends to do before he dies. That depends on his inner wisdom. Then he can complete his legacy or not, as he chooses. We will support whatever choice he makes. Aaron's legacy will be unique in that he is a member of this community who has been absent, which is the reason that we would like him to live with us for a while and to receive the transmission when he feels ready."

Aaron's expression reveals that he is overcome again, but differently. "You're saying that I belong here?"

"Yes. That both of you belong here."

This time, it is Rafa whose tears flow, and all three who embrace.

9

Immersion

Yuko-Hyun extends her hand stiffly. She is younger, twenty years to Parvati's thirty or so, and seems shy of Rafa. Aaron takes in her symmetrical, round face, short black hair, single-lidded eyes, and delicate frame. When she offers a deep bow, he realizes that she is deferring to what she sees as his great age.

Rafa says, shaking Yuko's hand awkwardly, "I'm Rafaela Aboulafia."

Aaron takes her hand in turn saying, "I'm Aaron Swanson."

"Excuse me, sir. May I ask why you don't have the same last name as your brother's unmarried daughter?" Aaron hears an accent in her carefully modulated voice and recognizes that she is a rare, recent immigrant. Considering her name, he infers that she is of Japanese and Korean descent. "Mom and Dad gave me her last name, and gave Eric his. May I ask where you were born?"

Yuko-Hyun's eyes narrow; Aaron can feel her dislike of the question, and her impulse to generalize that dislike to him.

Parvati exchanges a quick glance with Aaron and says, "That is a very long and important story that Yukie should share with you when she feels the time is right. It would be better to go to the school now, so that she can give you a tour of the building before our students return from their agro practica. Would that be all right with everyone?"

Rafa, apparently relieved to meet someone her own age,

attaches herself to Yuko-Hyun, and Parvati leads Aaron out of the garden through the nearest net gate onto the east path that leads north from the lodge. As Parvati carefully secures the net door behind them, tying it to the wall in two places, Aaron sees a group of students near the center. Their behavior brings a smile to his face. They are no more than five or six years old, and focus alternately and intently on cutting and placing lilies in baskets and on jumping and dancing wildly in place. Parvati comes to stand beside him while Yuko-Hyun and Rafa ask questions of the children.

"Did your mother tell you that we designed a body curriculum based on her work?" Parvati asks.

"She mentioned it, but that was all."

"We teach awareness first and apply those skills in the development of understanding and perceptions. The children learn to hold an absorptive state of relaxed alertness and to gently form and increase the focus of their attention and concentration. When they lose focus, they enjoy their energy and flesh until they're ready to focus again. So that's five levels of the body—awareness, understanding, perceptions, energy, and flesh. With gardening, they engage interbeing and sensations as well. That's all seven levels in one."

Parvati leads Aaron along the mulched path between lines of bushes covered in red-orange rosehips to the hothouses, where she stops and says, "All members sustain fertile states—as per the founders' application of your mother's work—but Yukie is just learning."

"I'm most familiar with cure states. Mom could be fierce."

Parvati laughs, open-mouthed. "We hope to capture that in the enactments, and to learn from you how to create care and cure states."

"Tell me about the enactments."

Parvati calls to Yukie, "Will you show Rafaela the garden and the school building while I show Aaron the ropes course?"

"Yes, teacher."

"The enactments are theater pieces that transmit four formative periods in your mother's life—and yours—so that you can receive our story of your life and we can interact with our history and call on it as the need arises."

"How did you identify the formative periods? Through Sarah?"

"The creative team reviewed the comm archives and interviewed Sarah, Doug, and John under hypnosis. Then we looked for those periods that changed the course of our community. We are fortunate that you will be here to enrich the transmission and to speak up when you suspect a miss, or mistake."

"During the play?"

"Yes. The players can improvise lines on the spot as the one they portray."

"Good heavens!"

"And that's how we'll get to know you," Parvati teases.

"I'm not the playful type."

"I know. I hope you'll forgive me if I'm too familiar. In preparing the script, I got to feel as if I knew you."

"You scanned my archive?"

"Yes, and looked at ours."

"That is thorough," Aaron observes uncomfortably. "Is John here now?"

"Yes. He came out by train after the funeral, and he's been staying with his granddaughter Gina. She lives here with her consorts. John intended to pay for your train ticket, and to take you along, but it seems that he was lost in grief and acted too slowly."

"I left abruptly. I have to confess that I was disturbed when he showed up. I'd forgotten all about him. I don't recall Mom mentioning him, and suddenly there he was sitting on her bed like the most important person in her life."

"Your Mother and John intended to spare their families. But that doesn't really work, does it?"

"Apparently not."

"The work they did together is a key aspect of our history."

"I see."

"That could be quite confronting for you," Parvati says tentatively.

"Yes. I'll do the best I can."

"You must feel free to speak out whenever something feels wrong. We don't draw a line between our inner and outer work. We conceal nothing—except for certain concepto guilders. We are still finding the line between privacy and secrecy in consort practice and human fertility."

"Are you—do you belong to that guild, to concepto?"

"I took the usual training, but I'm celibate and a teacher, like Sarah."

"Celibate? Here?"

"The majority of us live as celibates, or as solitaries who express sexuality without a consort or set of consorts."

"Set of consorts? Go slow, please. I muddled through celibacy without instruction, and haven't spoken of my flesh for years except to let others know that I was … unavailable."

"Here, you can ask anything, anytime. We speak openly— except with the uninitiated, like Rafaela—another exception," Parvati laughs. "We teach children about sexuality through a series of teaching initiations and rites. We can talk more at lunch. For now, we should focus on the school."

"Yes, of course." Aaron feels her discomfort and wonders, with a frisson of anxious desire, if she feels the same sharp urge to end her celibacy so as to join with him in body and being. The thought of it carries him away into fantasy. His heart pounds; his breath accelerates. It is with difficulty that he grounds his awareness, relaxes his flesh, and returns his focus to the schoolyard that they are approaching.

"Will you conceal things from Rafa and me?"

Parvati smiles. "Our intention is to reveal things gradually and fully by the end of the enactments. We planned to go step by step, as we do with fertility students and other guests, but I can see that won't work. Please be a patient partner as we figure it out."

"I'll do my best." He smiles, half hopeful that she feels and intends more than she is ready to reveal. "Tell me about the garden and hothouses."

Parvati leads Aaron into a hothouse and tells him that the agro guilders grow flowers as well as vegetables for canning. They pause to enjoy the fragrant bouquet of bay, basil, and other herbs, and the color bursts of various strains of heirloom tomatoes, peppers, eggplants, squash, and other fruits and flavorings that thrive year-round in the hothouses.

Then they make a short detour into the forest to look at the seven-sided glass and-cedar-walled sanctuary. The forest around it, which has grown far higher than when Aaron was last here, embraces garden seating that surrounds the sanctuary.

"It looks like a theater around a campfire."

"A gathering place for sacred rituals centered on Sarah's flame."

"And when that flame goes out ... "

"It won't if we let its source live in us."

"Source?"

"Our love and care of—and faith in—the foreground of God, the body of life."

Parvati turns to Aaron, beams, and gestures for him to follow her. He is transfixed by the spirit of this Eve in this garden, enamored of her sparkling eyes, full dark cheeks, and embodiment of fertility. He tries to return his attention to the campus. Through the forest on his right, he glimpses clusters of high tree houses, and ahead the forest theater with its living, white wall of white fungus-coated alder trees, beyond which rises a steep slope leading up to a craggy peak. A new structure stands below the crag; it resembles the forest sanctuary in having front walls of glass that make it nearly transparent—when they're not reflecting the sun's rays.

He points to it and asks, "Is that a new retreat center?"

"No. The original fertility and solitary retreat cabins are still on the other side of the peak. The new building is the memorial center."

"For funerals?"

"For remembering, honoring, and mourning what is lost."

"There seem to be gaps in the forest below."

"The fertility lodge is below and left of the peak, along with hot springs and guild housing and the habitat restoration center. We call that campus concepto because they conceive of ways to nurture life."

As she sees that he is about to ask a question, she says, "We will visit it later. Now, let's visit the theater." When they reach its living walls, she disappears into one of the narrow openings in the oval of trees. Aaron follows her through a diagonal tunnel, over a short bridge, and through a gap in a hard earth wall that is chest high. He sees that they are at the rear of the theater, and at the top of a slope into which has been built an amphitheater of U-shaped banks of seating. At the bottom is an oval thrust stage. Behind the stage is a wooden scrim; the scrim and stage are riddled with traps. Above is a bamboo frame to which solar lamps are affixed.

Aaron says, "This looks like a sanctuary."

"Yes, here, too, we encounter the liminal boundary of light and dark and keep in mind our sacred purpose. But we try to bring our best selves to the sanctuary, and here we come as we are."

"Wouldn't you want to meet God as you are?"

Parvati laughs. "We yogis are strivers, like our Sramana forebears. We value becoming over being and doing."

"Are you Hindu?"

"I am a Hindu sadhvi, which is like a nun except that we can take consorts and practice union as long as we still dedicate the whole of our lives to God."

"I'm glad to hear it."

"In my case there's a catch," she says lightly. "My family insists on a Hindu wedding."

"You practice endogamy? Like Jews?" he asks shyly.

She looks at him in surprise. "Yes. *They* do."

Rafaela stands on the south side of the basketball and tennis courts behind the school, toying with their fiber mesh enclosure. The under-thirteens—all clad in the same sunflower-colored shirt and denim overalls as the teachers—have just returned early from the agro center west of the school, where they were caring for animal buddies. Now they are playing a vigorous game of bike polo to embody the laws of mechanics that they have been learning for the past few months. Yukie is engaging the under-eighteens in teaching bike polo physics, and also supervising the under-sevens who are playing with the life-sized chess set or jumping rope with long plaits of bark that form standing waves as they snap and resonate like whips. Rafa notices that the children say little to each other, as if they know one another's minds.

South of the courts stands the schoolhouse that Yukie designed as her initiation project, which the students will be presenting to Rafa and *Tío* when he and Parvati arrive. Rafa has been enjoying the kinetic nature of the school and watching what Yukie does. Yet while Rafa has felt drawn to one vocation after the other—first to trading, and then to restoration, and then to designing and building structures—she is not drawn to teaching children. She decides to look at the forest north of the school, skipping around the courts to release the energy that has flooded into her from the students.

When she rounds the corner, she stops and stares at the forest, stunned. She hadn't noticed the shallow clearing lined with dangling ropes hanging from tree limbs, or the wood and fiber platforms and walkways that rise to the canopy and extend into the forest. It is a ropes course, a huge one that sends Rafa back to the last time she saw Mitzi and to each and every one of the last times that she saw one of the fallen angels who were their companions. Rafa runs away, going faster and faster until she rounds the far corner of the schoolhouse; there, she falls to her haunches against the living wall and buries her head between her knees. She wraps her hands over her head and rocks, trying in vain to relax and return to the morning.

She feels someone sit beside her and looks up, ready to run or attack.

"What happened?" Yukie asks calmly.

Rafa nestles her head in Yukie's lap, and Yukie rests a palm on Rafa's crown. Soon Rafa relaxes, and draws a deliberate but halting breath. Once she starts talking, she can't seem to stop until she has come to the very last day, when she left her old life behind. Yukie is patient. After a time, she understands about the ropes course and says, "You have to get up there soon. You can't let that define you."

"Easy for you to say."

"No, it isn't. Not for me."

"What do you mean?" Rafa asks suspiciously.

"I came from—I was born to a Korean father and Japanese mother in Okinawa, and we went to Korea to live in Seoul and pretend to be pure Korean, but then Seoul burned in the great fire and we fled to China, and then that burned, and we came here. My family had to move to Fulford to get me in here—Sarah finds it hard to refuse townies. You have no idea how lucky you are to have been born into it. They can't refuse you either."

Rafa stares at her appraisingly and asks incredulously, "How am I lucky?"

"Cascadia has thousands of places trying to prevent extinction, but this is the only experimental community that teaches fertility and restoration in a way that joins science and spirit, and that may be able to catalyze a renascence of medicine—with the help of your uncle. It's our species'—our world's—last and best hope."

"Medicine?"

"It started on the island of Kos in ancient times and lost its soul in modern times. Melissa and John brought it back like no one else."

"I don't know anything about that."

"You know more than you think you do. You sacrificed your first life to cure Denver of that demon. You know all you need to know."

"I had a terrible education. We sat and stared at screens. We never did anything real."

"My education was like that before I came here. All you have to do to catch up is find a real problem and solve it—and gather a support team who can tell you what you need to know and help you figure out what to do."

A bell rings loudly from the direction of the lodge. Yukie jumps up and says, "Help me get the students to the lodge."

"What is it?"

"The bear bell. Quick!"

Rafa's sense of peril grips her unpleasantly. She struggles to relax as she and Yukie and the older children gather the younger ones and move towards the lodge. Rafa and Yukie follow the smallest children to its back door. Yukie does a head count as they run. Soon they are sitting in the common room, where a large crowd has gathered, and is extending into the dining room.

The room falls silent as a lean, muscular young man dressed in black, shiny cowhide and long, sable-colored braids enters; he kneels beside Sarah in a position like that taken by runners at the beginning of a race. His face is smeared with black and red pigment. Rafa assumes that the young man is a performance guilder until he says to Sarah, "Grizzly!"

A man in a white chef's hat bolts into the common room from the kitchen holding a cleaver. A breathless woman in green enters the side door with a man in green following quickly behind.

"Ask what you will, Dirk," Sarah says calmly.

"Can we transport the grizzly alive?" Dirk, the kneeling warrior, asks loudly.

The man in green says, "The truck batteries are low, but we could rig a boat."

Dirk asks loudly, "Can we use the bear's meat?"

The chef says, "We can use the flesh of any forager—provided it tests pure."

"Can the web of life spare the bear?" Dirk asks.

The woman in green says, "Yes. We can compensate for his loss by spreading salmon heads, bones, and berry seeds in the forest. Plus sacrificing him would ease our restoration of the island's salmon runs."

Sarah asks formally, "Will anyone speak for the bear's life?"

"I will," says Dirk. "She is fierce and fine and filled with vitality. She could bear strong cubs and fertilize the forest for years before giving it her remains."

"Will anyone speak against the bear's life?"

"I will," Dirk speaks up again. "She came almost as far as the school, and may come again."

"What should we do?"

"Tranquilize, sacrifice, and slaughter the bear to protect the community."

"Let it be as you say, warrior," Sarah says. "Let this bear initiate you."

The young man stands and—to Rafa's shock—points straight at her, saying peremptorily, "You! Come with me."

"Can you take me in her place?" Aaron asks protectively from the dining room.

"No!" Dirk replies, fiercely.

Rafa's chest tightens. Barely able to breathe, she rises as if dreaming and follows Dirk, who has already exited and rounded the corner of the lodge heading north. Rafa races to catch up, succeeding as Dirk reaches the north edge of the garden. By the time they reach the schoolhouse, she is alert and alarmed and chilled to the bone. As they continue past the school to a forest trail and then to a clearing where five men in the same black gear and braids are waiting, it dawns on Rafa that he is literally running toward unknown danger.

As if reading her thoughts, an older man with broad cheekbones, raven-black hair, a round face, and an eagle feather in each braid points to Rafa and says ferociously, "Stop! She does not belong here!"

Dirk stops and kneels in the ritual pose he used before. "Doug says there are no warriors where Rafa comes from. She can bear witness to our ways, and she's tall and strong enough to help lift the bear."

"You're showing off. You're disrespecting the bear and the guild."

"Shall I take her back, Oke Ten?"

Oke Ten pauses and gazes into Rafa's eyes. "Have you any forest blood?"

Rafa's mind races, "My father's mother has roots in the forests of the far north, and my mother in the valley of the Riviera Maya."

"Your initiation?"

"None yet."

The man's stern face opens in consternation. "None?"

"I have yet to choose one."

"You have yet to earn one!"

Oke Ten spits into a clump of grass at the edge of the clearing, mutters something under his breath, and motions for Dirk to lead Rafa and the men up the forest path. It dawns on Rafa that she is still a child. Her wave of embarrassment is stopped short by a crash and a growl twenty yards on. Dirk stops abruptly. Rafa nearly runs into him, and then follows his eyes up to a red bag that is dangling from a high branch over a bear twice her height. The bear stretches up and sweeps at the bag with a massive paw that has long dark claws. Unsuccessful, she tries again and again. Dirk raises a black gun with both hands and takes careful aim. When he squeezes the trigger, Rafa hears a fleeting, high-pitched hiss. The bear continues to leap, eventually slicing the bag with her claws and catching a piece of fish in her jaws. Rafa thinks Dirk has missed, but as they wait and watch, the animal slows down. Her great head sinks to the left and her claws go limp. She falls to the ground like a great, heavy corpse.

Rafa takes a step forward, but Dirk puts up an arm and bars the way. She waits and watches and spots a dart sticking out of the bear's shoulder.

Dirk replaces the dart gun in a holster and draws a different sidearm. He holds it between his palms and creeps forward while the other men fan out behind him. Rafa follows at several paces, and soon hears a small explosion. Peering around the men, she sees blood trickling from a hole in the bear's head and feels a tremendous heave of sadness. There is no way to take that bullet back. She sees the others kneeling and joins them as Dirk recites what sounds like a rite or prayer in an unfamiliar language. Rafa inhales, only then realizing that she was terrified.

The group sets to work quickly and wordlessly. Dirk takes the lead, gesturing to the others to form a perimeter around the carcass. Rafa stands at the head where she can see everything as each man takes out a knife and begins to skin the flesh and butcher the meat. She asks, "How much does she weigh?"

Dirk says tersely, "Later."

Rafa watches as a warrior takes a large cut from the back and lifts it toward Rafa. She reaches under it, cradling its slippery undersurface. It is heavy and warm. She follows another young man with an armful of flesh who runs toward the lodge. She has been party to a killing, and feels a strange sense of lost innocence. "What kind of fertility center is this," Rafa mutters bitterly. As the bear's flesh drags her down, she struggles to finish well and prove herself equal to the task. Her exertion is so great that when she reaches the lodge, she barely notices that the common room and dining room have emptied.

Even so, when she pushes the swinging door into the kitchen, Rafa is struck by the density of wall and ceiling storage, especially above, where so many items are hanging from hooks attached to the ceiling grid that at first glance they appear to form the ceiling. She dashes under it after the young man and the chef, who run through another swinging door in the far wall. To her surprise, it leads to the top landing of a long oval staircase. The sounds of their footsteps are like an out-of-tune steel drum, and the air grows colder below the deep-welled windows as they descend into an ice cellar beneath the path south of the lodge.

She is too distracted now to think of pain, but in her exhaustion bumps into the metal wall that is backed by a melting array of ice blocks, and stumbles on the central floor drain that must let out above or at the orchards below.

"Tell them to send the fat and the sirloin first," the chef says to the warrior. "There's just enough time to test the meat and—if it's clean—marinate it for Dirk's initiation feast tonight."

As the young man clangs up the stairs, Rafa holds the bear meat up so that the chef can slide a net around it and take the weight of it; then she catches the corners of the square net with a hook. Together, they hang the cut from a ceiling rail, and Rafa stands back, her clothes streaked with blood, to gape at the dangling sides of beef and goat and an array of cured meats.

"Where'd you get the ice?" she asks, panting.

"Mount Washington—the big island. We still have winter."

"We're having it for dinner?" she asks dubiously, thinking of the living beast.

"I've been waiting for this day," the chef answers brightly, opening a drawer and pulling out a box marked "meat test kit". "Dirk has been ready for months."

"That's so … fast."

"Unlike you." The chef reaches for a towel and tosses it to Rafa. "Get going! Bear fat spoils fast."

As another warrior comes rushing down the stairs, Rafa nods, shakes out her arms, wipes the blood away, and tucks the towel into her waistband. She spends the next hour working with the warriors in relay according to Dirk's silent instructions. Soon, nothing remains in the clearing but hide and men, at which point Oke Ten says kindly, "Go to the lodge, now. You can attend tonight's rite."

When Rafa enters the lodge, she finds Aaron waiting in the common room with a towel and a set of clean green clothes of the kind worn by many of the residents. Rafa follows her *tío* upstairs to the cell where she will be staying. She sheds her clothes carefully on the polished bamboo flooring, avoiding the narrow bed, bedside rug, armoire, desk, and chair. Then she puts on a towel and follows Aaron to the back porch and the bathhouse to its right.

An hour later, Aaron and Rafa enter the dining room for the midday dinner. Sarah guides them through the buffet and on to a table beside the monumental fireplace, where they sit down with Doug, Parvati, and Yuko-Hyun to enjoy a meal of eggs, venison sausage, hardtack, and fruit compote. At first, Rafa is ravenous and relaxed and beginning to feel at home, and glad to join in the chorus of conversation filling the large yet cozy room. But soon small children begin to gather around them, to touch her clothes and to watch and listen. Seeing a preschooler casually pleasure herself, Rafa feels a surge of discomfort. Parvati draws the child aside and gives her the choice to respect others by going to her room or by stopping; the child stops placidly. Yuko-Hyun asks Rafa about her sexual initiation, and she confesses that she had none.

Rafa reminds herself to relax into local manners and mores, and to align her state with those who are used to them. As the meal draws her energy down and her breathing becomes loose and easy, Yoko-Hyun and *Tío* draw Rafa into a discussion of the history of North American experiments in intentional community. Rafa wants to know more about the Catholic settlements at Ville-Marie, and the Protestant experiments at Plymouth, Dorchester, and Brooke Farm, as well as the Ebenezer Colony that became the Amanas. She wants to examine the archives for information on Moravians, Friends, Mennonites, Mormons, Congregationalists, and Unitarians. To be without history would be to ride blind into the snares of the subconscious, to miss the chance of knowing her place in the body of life in time. She thinks of choosing history as a vocation, but here each person keeps the history of the species in the way that her Jewish relations kept that of their tribe.

After lunch, Yuko-Hyun takes Rafa and *Tío* down to the fabro center to meet Björn, who will give them a tour. At the bottom of forest path to the fabro-yard, before she goes up to the school, Yuko-Hyun points out a huge bear of a man with tousled blond hair, broad shoulders, and big hands. Rafa watches him carefully to see if she, like Yuko-Hyun, would choose Björn as a mentor. He moves quickly, confidently, and energetically. She guesses that he loves both his work and his workers.

Aaron shakes Björn's strong hand and recounts meeting Björn's father on his previous visit to the community. Aaron remarks on the Australian accent that Björn has maintained despite never having visited his parents' country. He replies in a booming baritone, "They died in the Great Poisoning. Hard drinkers, they were. The other Aussies took me in and taught me to speak English properly." He winks at Rafa and says, "I heard you're going to become a trader."

"Right now, I'm thinking about fabro."

Björn raises an eyebrow skeptically, and moves directly into the role of tour guide. He begins with the fabro yard, pointing out the main features from the edge of its sand-covered clearing. These include several widely-separated mounds of metal and earth, pitted and scorched and caked with soot, fenced about to keep animals and children from venturing too close. The nearest he names as the "Viking Steel Forge." A fabro guilder in a grey uniform is crouched in front of it, feeding its maw with scoops of charcoal. Behind her, Rafa sees a bellows, anvil, sledgehammer, and bucket of metal shards. The mound beyond the forge is the glassblowing oven.

At the end of the clearing, beyond all the mounds, sits a long structure that joins what was once a series of buildings. The near wall is comprised of hanging panels, one of which has been pushed aside to reveal a large production room. In its center, a team of fabro guilders is riveting metal rods to make a large, light framework that will become a shed roof. Around the perimeter of the production room stand floor pens filled to overflowing with raw materials: scavenged metal scraps, glass shards, shims and blocks of wood, sand, pea gravel, plastic bottles, clay, and broken pottery. Above the pens hang rows of crates filled with pinecones, sticks, moss, and charcoal.

Rope and pulley rigging rises from the floor to the ceiling and then through an opening in the roof to a set of pylons. The rigging continues on a row of pylons that march up the side of the mountain and out of sight. A team of guilders is securing a molded spa pool to the rigging, presumably in preparation for hauling it up to the road for transport by tractor.

"Everything looks like scrap," Rafa says.

"I heard that," Björn says amiably as he sweeps his visitors toward the nearest mound. "This looks a pile of rubbish but it's a Viking forge. You've got roots in Sweden, haven't you, Aaron?"

"I do. But isn't steel production very energy-intensive?" Aaron asks.

"We use it to make knives and construction frames, and we don't make many. But you're right; the little charcoal we make and use burns through our carbon budget like wildfire." Björn leads them to the weathered mound of clay and ore and adds, "Let's have a look, then."

He asks the woman in gray to demonstrate the bellows, and turns back an oilcloth to reveal the anvil and the sledgehammers that he calls "sledgies." He tells with gusto the tale of his pilgrimage to the Great Lakes to apprentice with a blacksmith who made a hobby and then a business of recreating Viking swords. Björn picks up a discarded piece of scrap metal and says, "Nothing wasted, nothing wanting."

Björn leads his guests to the fence around the next mound, where they see a steel-walled oven. A woman with shaved temples is showing a group of leather-aproned fabro guilders how to mold glass. Björn nods to her to continue and says to Aaron, "We like our glass panels, and we have the know-how to make fused, molded, and blown glass."

"That must take a lot of fuel, too," Aaron says.

Folding his arms over his chest, Björn shifts his weight to one leg. "We haven't worked out the whole equation. Making charcoal is quite an art. If we make it too often, we lose sustainability; if we don't make it often enough, we lose skills. Tricky, that."

Next, Björn strides across the fabro yard, past several other mounds, to the shed; he pushes open the rest of the door panels to reveal its hangar-like interior. Rafa and Aaron catch him up; Aaron says, "I made a bookshelf at school."

"And it was level and plumb?"

"No!" *Tío* laughs. "But I used it anyway."

Björn says with a chortle, "You'll get no points for that here, mate."

They watch the fabro workers for a time, and then enter and pass the pens of raw materials. When they reach the far wall, Björn slides open a large door and leads them into and through a hallway. They pass a room on the left that is dedicated to communications devices; Aaron stops to look in through its door. Peeking over his shoulder, Rafa sees a worktable, a wall covered by tools on pegs, and shelves filled with old devices. Björn enters and opens a huge map drawer in the worktable to pull out several large sheets of hemp paper; he places them on top of the table. "These are the plans for our early warning systems for earthquakes and storms and predators. We have devices in place and want to expand our circuits, but we've run into compatibility issues. We could use your advice."

"I'd be delighted to do whatever I can."

Björn leaves the papers where they are. "Right-o. I'll hold you to it, then."

Afterwards, Björn leads them on down the hall past specialty rooms and through a sliding door into a large shed with a huge, two-story loom. "This is soft fabro. We make fibers of hemp, wool, bark, bamboo, and flax. The crafters have begun weaving sheets and blankets on this loom. After the spring equinox, when the light is good in here, they'll re-warp the loom for shirting."

"Do you weave all the cloth here?" Rafa asks.

"All but the cloth that people bring here when they arrive or trade."

"I'm amazed," Aaron says. "Your cloth is finer than Amana cloth, and your colors are true and vivid! Parvati's shirt looks like a bouquet of marigolds."

"Parvati chooses the colors. Her family knows the India trade back to front. We buy dyes from them, and she gets us the fair price."

"Where do you make your wine?"

"We stopped making it a long time back. We're sober, now, except for Doug; true blue incorrigible, that one. But we still have orchards and vines at the bottom of the hill, and the agro guild will soon be pressing cider and juice."

Björn goes on through a door in the far wall, which opens into a low room filled with over two dozen fabro workers in small groups who are practicing fiber arts such as knitting, quilting, rug-making, and basketry. Rafa smells coffee and hears strands of newsy gossip.

"No story today?" Björn asks the room.

A white-haired woman sitting at his elbow replies without looking up from her quilt stitching. "We're between stories, Björn. How about a saga?"

"Best hold that for Aaron's enactments."

"We've heard about that saga," she says, tipping her head toward Aaron. "And made costumes and props for it."

Rafa laughs. "Why does everyone know more about his plans than we do?"

"Small world, mate," Björn replies, "smaller than a small town. You want to know anything, ask anyone."

Björn winks, and watches Aaron speak with a man who is making coffee, a group of young people who are knitting winter sweaters for schoolers, and a group of white-haired women who are working on quilt squares. "Are those for the memorial room?"

"Yes," says a woman with very sparse hair.

"Each is for a habitat," says a young woman, "Mine is for the one south of Juyong, the pass in China, where a sandstorm nearly buried Yuko-Hyun."

Aaron looks at Rafa and says somberly, "I can't even imagine it."

"She could hardly talk when she arrived," Björn says, "but concepto treated her energy body and helped her come right."

Rafa makes a mental note to go to concepto and to ask for the same treatment.

10

Dirk's Initiation

For Sarah, waking up from her daily siesta is like emerging from a deep pool in a dark cave. Today, she dreamt she was lying beside Melissa, looking at the living and loving them and yet relieved to be free of the burden of caring for them. As she sits and breathes, light and life fill her flesh. It hurts at first, and then she uses the aches and pains as guides to the work ahead, work that she hopes will fulfill her friendship group's chosen destiny. After a few more breaths, she feels the joy of looking to the horizon beyond modern rapacity to a time when humanity will craft its essential role in the body of life.

She sighs. If Melissa had not been stubborn to the end, their coming rebirth would have been easier, but having Aaron and Rafa with them is more wonderful than she could have hoped. Between them, they carry enough shadow to be primed to turn it into light, and so to become engines in the loving renewal of a death-obsessed, war-soaked world. Aaron already sees the resilience of evolved generative life; Rafa will soon learn to join the material and ethereal, and—with grace—illuminate the way forward for her part in humanity's urgent cultural evolution.

Sarah stirs her bones and, letting her legs dangle over the side of the bed, turns every particle of her being to the light. Taking up her cane, she dresses and descends the stairs to enjoy afternoon tea with Rafa and Aaron. By the time she reaches the small sitting room at the northeast corner of the ground level of the lodge, she has resolved to take them on a tour of concepto right away. Their burden of time debts is too great to take the risk of being careless of their fertility. If she goes about it right, she will share her vision of an exuberant new phase of human metamorphosis possible in this wilding haven. They can then adapt and develop it, and—with luck—see through and beyond it.

It is a tricky business; if they were ordinary guests, she would simply invite them to respect and share their way of life; but to these guests, she must reveal as much light and shadow as she can so as to enable them to see the way of life that was and that may still be. The problem is that she never saw as far as the founders. Now that they are all gone, the community has run past its visions, and the kindred is running away from an unacceptable past rather than toward a brighter future. It took Sarah too long to realize that the founders had simply run with part of Melissa's vision, the greater part perhaps, and it had taken Melissa too long to accept that her embodied experience might still—directly or indirectly—complete the work of their generation.

Entering the sitting room, Sarah goes to the east-facing window to regard the hill that rises half a mile north of the lodge. As she reflects on how vast it had seemed at first, and how small it seems now, she hears Aaron's voice behind her say, "Good afternoon." When he comes to stand beside her, she says, "I like to tell the children that this land is our beloved sleeping queen. The dark gray columns on top of the hill form her crown, the forested slopes her hair and robes, and the cabins and terraced gardens her jewels. I tell the children that the founders transformed the modern urge for death into an urge for life, and that they have entrusted us with doing that for the queen."

"I'm not much for personification." He laughs ruefully.

"Ah. And imagination?" she teases.

"My parents taught me to observe the world the way it is, to explore phenomena with an open mind, to test them continually and with as few preconceived notions as possible. I'm a scientist, I suppose; an empiricist."

"You'll be a good guide to Rafa as she structures her being and learns to penetrate the unknown and discover the new."

"Imagination can be treacherous."

"Like any tool; use it at your own risk for your own purpose," Sarah replies pointedly. Then she turns and takes Aaron's arm and starts toward the tea table. "With a nice hot cup of tea."

They see that Rafa has already prepared the tea tray and put it on the table; she is ready to pour. After they are comfortably seated, Sarah quietly introduces the topic of fertility. She knows that Melissa did not like the community's spiritual smörgåsbord or their practice of union; she also knows that Aaron and Rafaela have both struggled with fertility, Aaron in sad celibacy and Rafa with injurious profanity. Sarah is certain that the concepto guilders would know just how to help these guests if they had come as students or clients, but they didn't. Moreover, the transmission is designed for initiates. A tour and discussion will allow Sarah to judge how best to mesh their guests' views with the demands of the legacy project and the ethics of the community.

"We are asking you to adapt very quickly, and I know that it could be overwhelming. That's the reason that I'd like to introduce you to the concepto center and to the fertility guilders. They use interactive dialogue to open body and being to fertile states. Those are different from your care states; they catalyze becoming—they invite ceaseless transformation. Their counseling patterns personal integration and transformation for the purpose of forming thirds, which are the potentials that come into being in any deep encounter."

"I don't know what that 'thirds' means," Rafa says tensely.

"When two people come together, a potential forms. For our students, it may lead—through consort practice—to a child. For our members, it may—depending on the situation—lead to an initiation project, a vocational initiation, a lifework, or a legacy."

"Can we think about it?" Rafa asks guardedly.

"Yes, of course. But it's only a matter of time before you learn the hard way that consulting with a fertility guilder can save you time, pain, and trouble."

"How can you be so sure?" Rafa asks.

"We've been counseling newcomers for over forty years, and it becomes more important as our rate of change increases. In fact, we've gotten ahead of ourselves!" Sarah chuckles. "We've dropped and missed things on the way, and have to go back and try and pick them up."

"Through enactments?" Aaron asks.

"Yes, that's one way."

"We should prepare for those. Let's go to concepto," Aaron says to Rafa.

Sarah then turns the conversation to lighter topics and, once they've finished their tea, leads them outside and along the east path to the front door of the concepto lodge, which is a smaller copy of the main one. She points out the bamboo farm to the north of the building that doubles as a Zen garden, the hot springs pools that accommodate groups, and the nearby cabins that some fertility students use for specialized practices. Rather than casually describing what those might be, she says, "Do speak up any time you feel uncomfortable for any reason, or have questions."

Rafa confesses, "I should tell you that I heard a lot of rumors on the way—that you enchant people and then take advantage of them."

Sarah shakes her head. "That excuse is as old as infidelity! When students arrive, we make it clear that they are fully responsible for their own actions. Most aren't used to it. Some adopt our worldview and choose surrogate therapy or other practices that they can't integrate on returning home. Those may abrogate responsibility after the fact." Sarah pauses and continues thoughtfully, "Which reminds me to say that we invite our students—and you—to use what your grandma called transference. That is, you can rely or depend on us—with the expectation that you will assume responsibility and authority for your actions as soon as you are able."

Aaron asks Rafa solicitously, "Are you ready to go inside?"

"Always and never," Rafa replies with a crooked smile.

Sarah takes Aaron's left arm and Rafa's right, and asks tenderly, "Would you like to meet the guilder who's teaching celibacy practice today?"

Aaron says ironically, "I'd rather move on to the role of blushing virgin."

Rafa is astonished. "You're a virgin? Ridiculous! Incredulous!"

"I wasn't at your age, but I am now," Aaron smiles shyly. "Seeing the forest coming to life again inspires me to try the same thing."

Sarah's eyes smile as they pass over the threshold of the concepto lodge. Lifted by the energy of her younger companions, she slips easily into the envelope of bliss created and sustained by the fertility guild. When she feels her guests respond to it, she sheds a burden of care. They have the natural gifts—and some of the skills—to use the enactments for initiation and for legacy creation. Sarah laughs with joy when Aaron expresses his awareness by saying, "This structure feels like a tree of life that joins earth and sky."

Rafa says warily, "It's what you feel before a revival preacher or guru siphons off your energy or your money."

For a moment, the ground beneath Sarah's feet seems to open into a dark realm of restless ghosts. She shifts her continuous practice by taking that darkness in on her in breath and breathing out pure joy. "You recognize the energy rightly," she says after a pause, "but we can teach you—as we do all students—to turn dark into light, bad into good, despair into joy."

"You mean take energy from others."

"Not at all. I mean to turn obstacles into opportunities, and to share those consciously and effectively."

Rafa does not reply, but Sarah can tell that Rafa is paying close attention as Sarah describes the images in the molded glass panels of the entry foyer, which represent the bodies of their habitats and biome. Sarah also notes that Rafa is more curious and less guarded when they enter the hallway and pause by a door to listen to a chant master teaching a blessing. At the next door, Rafa looks in through the window as Sarah points out groups of couples who are learning to use seven aspects of the body to enhance fertility.

"What if they don't conceive a child?" Aaron asks.

"Some go to a modern clinic for treatment, but most choose to adopt a habitat."

Sarah leads them as far as a pair of gauzy curtains and says, "The rooms on the other side of the curtain are for individual bodywork and advanced consort practice. Disorders of the energy body, such as tenacious hell states, fractures, or deformations may interfere with inner or outer union."

Rafa says, "I want a treatment."

"I'll arrange it."

"Mom never talked about curing the energy body," Aaron says skeptically.

"Your parents sometimes sent us patients, but they tended to be fatalistic about diseases of the energy body."

"I didn't know that!" Aaron says with some distress.

Sarah says kindly, "Finding out things you didn't know gives you a chance to know your parents better."

"There will be more?"

"I sincerely hope that we will all know your mother better."

Aaron sighs. "Yes, of course."

As Sarah leads her companions back to the foyer and on up the stairs, Aaron says to Rafa, "Your grandparents tended to look backward. I think your dad did the same. I was free of it—a bit—by virtue of being the communicator."

"I like looking ahead," Rafa declares.

"You'll see more of the future as you gain perspective on your past and present," Sarah says.

Rafa frowns dubiously.

When they reach the landing of the third floor, Sarah asks Rafa to open the door to the hallway. Here, it is lined on either side by curtains rather than by walls. Those on the left are made of felted bark and those on the right of gauze. A breeze billows the curtains, releasing the scents of oranges and roses accented by cloves, clary sage, and other herbs and spices. Sarah pauses to inhale deeply; the others do the same. Then she motions for Aaron and Rafa to look through the gauzy curtains on their right.

She sees Rafa become aware that several couples beyond the curtain are nude and seated facing, gazing into each other's eyes, arms and legs wrapped around their partners. As she continues down the hall past rooms with more advanced students, Sarah feels Aaron respond with distress. She takes his arm and draws him gently back toward the front stair. Rafa follows.

When the hall door has closed behind them, Sarah asks, "Do you have any questions?"

"Why are some in groups?" Rafa demands.

"Our students can elect to practice union, in which case they can choose a single consort—or group of consorts—and commit to practicing with them."

"Do they get married?"

"They commit for a year. If all goes well and they wish to continue, they commit again for three years, and then five and ten. In the twentieth year, they are free to commit for life or not, using any rites they choose."

"Can you have same-sex partners?" Aaron asks.

"We divide students into groups by sexual expression—yes or no—and then by solitary practice—yes or no—and then by partner preference. The last is generally one of three types that we call simple-same, simple-diff, and complex-any."

"Sounds chaotic."

"We find it to be just the opposite. Members can enter into a partnership that is free of confusion or deceit—including self-deceit."

"So what groups could I choose from—if I became a student?" Rafa asks.

"You could be a celibate like me. We learn to reroute the circulation of our energy bodies to bypass the generative organs—which is very relaxing and energizing, not at all like the old ascetic way of overpowering the body."

"Or?"

"You could be a solitary, which means that you would

practice on your own—which is like masturbation except that we use a sacred practice."

"My mom brought me up to be Catholic. I can't even imagine that."

"We enhance integrity by combining spirituality and sexuality. Many Catholics do that now."

"What else?"

"You can choose to declare a partner preference. If you want a same-sex partner, and you expect to always want that, you declare as a simple-same."

"What if I always want a female partner?" Aaron asks.

"You would declare as a simple-diff."

"You said there were three main categories," Aaron prompts.

"Fertility guilders who want to pattern the sexual habits of others declare as complex-any. Those who initiate students learn to read the body and being of any partner, discern how that partner can best express arousal and union, and complement the partner's expression so as to engage in a first and only union or partial union."

Aaron smiles. "So they're ... sexual gourmets?"

"Their vocation is transmitted by an arduous series of courses and sustained by detailed sacred vows. We view it as our highest art, and our way of leading and patterning restoration."

Aaron frowns. "That sounds triumphalist."

"We do our utmost to care for and to cure the body of life. In that sense we are competitive—but we are also cooperative, collaborative, and collusive."

"Wow," Rafa says pensively, "no wonder people don't get it."

"It will take a while to integrate all of this," Aaron agrees. "How long until the first enactment?"

"That's up to you."

"Whew," Aaron smiles. "You sure know how to put on the pressure."

"We like to think that we create a crucible for change—but do let us know if it gets to be too much, and we'll slow it down. You're strivers. It's key that you find your own paces and avoid pushing yourselves too hard."

Doug has never been so glad to spend time with John. In recent years, their conversations have been few and superficial. Now that they and Sarah are the only ones still standing, this chance to delve into their early years of independence is precious and momentous. Doug wishes that John and Sarah were stronger; their waning vitality and Melissa's death fill his heart with regret that they did not meet more often. He loves them like crazy and wants to be strong for them, which is one reason he is pushing himself to remain a sassy Devil's advocate when he would prefer to cry in his scotch.

Dirk's feast distracts them all, and gives them a chance to relax the responsibilities of sage elderhood and to have a blast— to the extent that they are able. Right now, Doug is watching Aaron watch Sarah amplify the drama of Dirk's feast. They are sitting at the head table that the hospitality guilders made of platforms and single tables, their backs to the south windows of the dining room. Doug feels like an Oxford Don watching a roomful of declaiming students for signs of promise. He would rather keep tabs on Rafa, who is showing new promise as she sits at the other end of the table with Dirk and his parents, just above his cohort of initiates and the elders of the warrior guild. Rafa may very well turn out to be the street-smart apprentice that Doug has been seeking for decades; he hopes that Björn or one of the others will not waste her talents on a lesser life work.

Sarah pressed him to take Dirk as an apprentice, but Dirk's famous charisma was lost on Doug, who couldn't protect him as well as the warrior guild from the desires and dreams of lovers, johns, and sexual conquistadors. Doug prefers Rafa's vibrant curiosity and common sense. She has the canny self-confidence to cut through any kind of charm or drama, and the deflating and debunking speech that can strip away—or match—any pretense she meets. Plus, she has the generosity of mind and spirit and the commitment to the general good required for the win-win-win trades that Doug has perfected. He also has no need to keep up appearances with Rafa; she sees right through him.

Most people don't. Most people take Doug for a healthy seventy years or younger, and take it for granted that he will be trading indefinitely. Part of this comes of Doug's stories of being oversexed, but the truth is that he would rather get lucky in the bathroom than in the bedroom now, and while he pretends to enjoy great adventures on the open seas, he'd rather be here enjoying Sarah's warmth and the little luxuries that she provides for him—like having a fertility guilder trim his facial hair to prevent his nose looking like a stone-studded root ball, and arranging for a hospitality guilder to bring his dinner plate so that he doesn't reveal his encroaching infirmity by tipping the plate or by tripping and falling.

Doug will talk with Rafa later. For now, he enjoys Aaron's kind, open face and steady gaze, which misses nothing and discards nothing and—to Doug's eyes—reveals everything. Doug is fairly sure that he sees the exact moment when Aaron gets that Sarah is writing and directing the pageant of everyday life here, using festivals and rites to focus its energy and address its concerns.

Doug expects that by the time the curtains rise on the first enactment, Aaron will have worked out that Sarah's lines cue the continuing improvisation that creates this community, chooses its themes and character arcs, and thereby steers its course through the seas of space and time.

Doug is also watching John, who is looking into the distance. He was never a handsome man, but was always so well-liked and respected that many thought him attractive. Since his arrival, he has been looking more and more like his old self: his carriage tall and lean and upright, his white-fringed skull shapely, his late-growing nose finely sculpted, and his eyes deep and ocean green, framed rather than curtained by ample, crinkled lids.

Doug is likewise happy to talk with Aaron, who is coming alive here—so much so that Doug half believes that Sarah will succeed in persuading the son to fulfill his mother's promise. Doug is acutely aware of how destructively his generation lived in spite of all the dissenters and creatives among them, like himself and his friends. They made too many mistakes, were too enchanted by chips and crystals. When he thinks of the chemicals leaching into the water tables below California sand from the electronic devices he had once promoted, he wishes that he had sold crack instead. Better to hurry a few lost souls to the grave than to erase the future of life on earth.

At least Doug had fun paying his time debts. He loved leaving behind the role of venture capitalist to become a high-seas trader, and to co-found the traders' guild in doing so. His life consisted of one long series of adventures that made it possible for this community to restore the forests he loves, and that allowed him to keep and share the skin-of-the-teeth survival stories that help his older customers release their possessive individualism enough to cooperate on the big purchases.

The groups are the ones who buy barges, stud horses, and

high-quality wild game charcuterie. Even this community—where fewer personal goods signals greater integration and importance—buys enough big-ticket items to keep Doug at the top of his game and his guild happy. The nature of the community also keeps him happy; he and Cookie could have made a bundle on bear meat, but they would rather feast and share in the ceremony.

Thus, when the drum in the common room begins to beat steadily, Doug is out of his chair before any other elder to claim the first position by the stage where the warriors will enact their rite. When the rest of the diners have gathered behind Doug, filling the room with colorful clothing, sculptural hair stylings, and elaborate temporary tattoos, Doug grabs a young warrior and leans on him. The warrior rites are always long, as well as dramatic.

First, several elders commemorate Dirk's childhood and eulogize its end. Dirk's mentor then recounts the completion of Dirk's childhood purpose and his new membership in the adult community, and then announces his provisional entry into the guild. For the sake of formality and the benefit of their guests, an elder—Oke Ten—explains that Dirk will serve the guild as an initiate from the time when his marking is complete until he earns his vocation, defines his lifework, and achieves full membership. Dirk then swears to uphold the community mission of conscientiously restoring and protecting the web of life, and the guild mission of openly and safely bounding the community. Oke Ten then promises to mentor Dirk, which surprises Doug. Oke Ten takes few initiates; Doug wonders if he has taken Dirk under his wing for sake of his flaws or his gifts.

Then comes the drama that the children have been waiting so patiently to see. A warrior shaves Dirk's head and burns the clippings. A member of the craft arts guild scarifies and tattoos Dirk's upper arms, a process that will yield a subtle result that is suitable for an initiate, and leave room for a lifetime of accomplishments. When they finish, the performance guilders take up their instruments and feature Dirk in the sport entertainment, which focuses on fire juggling and acrobalancing.

Finally, when Doug's bladder is as full as it can get, Sarah concludes the rite by giving Dirk a pendant that will admit him to adults-only events. He then replies, "Thank you for this opportunity to give service." All present repeat the words with quiet sincerity. It had taken Doug years to set aside his clownish needling of initiates so as to fully enjoy that sacred moment of commitment.

Soon after, Doug sees Rafa pushing through the crowd. When she is close, she asks, "Do you think I should be a warrior or a fabricator?"

"I think you should be a trader. But it's your choice. Explore all your options."

"How?"

"I can give you a list of young people to talk to. I can also give you the name of a counselor."

As Dirk and the young people descend to the basement to dance, John watches Sarah remove a brooch that has been decorating her robe and will light their way with a tiny solar pinlight. He follows her out the east door and along the east path to a trail that passes the concepto clearing and continues straight on up the hill. After they have climbed slowly and with care for some time, pausing now and then to catch their breath, Sarah says with a touch of anxiety, "You've never been so quiet, John. It's like you're leaving us."

John does not want to talk about Melissa's death. He knows that Sarah wants to hear of it, to put Melissa to rest by hearing of the moment when her flesh turned cadaverous. He prefers to recall when her life left her body and joined his, but he does not want to talk of that for fear of losing touch with her, or of leaving behind his living friends. Finally he says, "I'm here and not here. My flesh is here; my awareness is with her."

"Melissa?"

"Yes."

"Are you reliving … the old days?"

"You could say that," he agrees reluctantly.

"What would you say?"

"The night she died, after Aaron left her side, I sat with her, and her spirit left her body and entered mine. It was like … a luminous living fire."

"I've heard of that," Sarah says gently.

"You have?"

"I didn't know that it could happen without long and intense preparation. You're fortunate."

"I think so, too," he says with a deep sigh.

Sarah asks hesitantly, "Did you—forgive the past?"

"It wasn't necessary. I raged all the way there—mostly at myself for leaving her seventy years ago, and for missing my second chances twenty and thirty years later. But when I took her hand, it was as if she had always been with me, and always would be. She talked a lot about you and Doug at the end, and regretted not coming here. The clinic, you know. She couldn't leave it. I don't know if you realize how much she loved you and Doug. She was quiet about it, but loved you deeply—as do I."

"Do you regret not marrying her when you had the chance?"

"I like to think we did the right thing. We faced consequences either way."

The silence between John and Sarah fills with unspoken feeling as they reach a fork in the trail and continue on a side trail toward the memorial. Soon Sarah's pinlight reveals the base of a wall, and she reaches up and pulls a door handle. As they enter, lights go on around the perimeters of both floor and ceiling. When the door closes behind them, Sarah touches a sensor in the wall. Rows of solar-enhanced light spreaders emit low light. "Is that enough light?"

"Yes. After the darkness, this little bit of light shows all."

"Come," Sarah says. She leads him up several levels to the back of the top level, where she stops and points upward to the huge quilt that extends the full width of the back wall.

"This is the memorial quilt. We have six or seven rows to go before we commemorate the habitats we lost in the modern age and that we are continuing to lose."

They gaze up at the quilt somberly. It's both beautiful and disturbing. Sarah begins to mutter prayers, and after a few minutes, John smiles. He can hear Melissa pointing out Sarah's easy relation to distant losses, and how it differs from his closer relation to death, which he gained through years of caring for the living and then companioning them through death and dying. He feels her laugh sharply, and asks Sarah in his sonorous, bracing voice, "Are you trying to cheer me up?"

Sarah looks at him in surprise. After a pause, they both chortle, and she says, "Sorry. We carry so much unexpressed grief, some of it from our students and other visitors. I don't know when to let it pass us by, and when to flip it so that it can push us gently onward."

John replies gently, "Put it in perspective. You're over ninety. You gave it your all—we all did. It's time to put your burden down. Those who come after will have to work it out for themselves anyhow."

"But they'll carry the time debts we didn't pay in addition to their own."

"You've taught them to earn credits, haven't you?"

Sarah sighs deeply. "Very sanguine! I always loved that about you."

"Even when you didn't like me?"

"That doesn't matter anymore," Sarah says with a playful smile. She turns and walks toward the wall of windows at the front. John follows her, descending carefully and pausing now and then to peer through the windows.

"I can't see lights below us—or anywhere!"

"The sanctuary is lit," Sarah says, pointing east of the lodge.

"Where's that?"

"Gina didn't show you? She and her wives go there often."

Sarah stops on the second level near the west wall, beside a single large piece of yellow cedar. Inset on either side of it are carved bas-reliefs of a staff entwined by a snake. On its flat front is a painted landscape inset with an ornately etched metal plaque. As John comes around to look at it, he sees that the painting incorporates a collage of photos and testimonials about Melissa and Dan and their family.

"My goodness! I haven't seen these pictures in years!" Stepping back, he hears Melissa wishing that she had looked better and at the same time pointing out the miseries the smiling faces did their best to conceal. John feels a pang. There is Melissa with Aaron. There is Eric before he came here, when he was still optimistic about his future and eager to go on to his next adventure. And there is the whole family—Melissa, Dan, Aaron, and Eric—standing confidently on telemark skis in the backcountry, probably behind Winter Park, which was close to Denver and a favorite winter getaway spot. In all of the photos, the family is in the foreground and John is absent. He knows that he has family albums just like this, filled with pictures of happy faces and family feeling and holidays and graduations that come once in a lifetime and tell who belongs and who doesn't. John can hardly stand to look at these; they show that he belonged to her psyche but not to her life. He says, with a click of the tongue, "I see it now. For me, these are time debts that should have been time credits."

Sarah takes him to another memorial dedicated to his own family. He knows that Sarah means to make things right by including both families, but he feels close to tears. Here are more time debts that should have been credits. He appeals to Melissa for comfort, but she is silent. As he masters his feelings with difficulty, it occurs to him that both memorials are out of place. "Why do you have these here, in this building?"

"I've been thinking that you and she must have been founders. We'd have no community—or a very different one—if you and Melissa hadn't done the work you did together."

"Do you see these as time credits?"

"Yes! Oh, yes."

Hear that Missy? Our sacrifices weren't for nothing— they were for this, whatever it is!

11

Initiates

Rafa leaves breakfast early, puts on a felted wool jacket, and steps out onto the muddy forest trail that leads from the lodge to the treehouses beyond the theater. She observes yellow, black, and spotted banana slugs keeping company with snails; moist snags feeding bright orange shelf fungi; a hawk soaring overhead that quiets the small birds in the trees; and a skunk cabbage withering in a gnat-infested depression full of leaf-stained water. At first, she took the forest for a tree farm and admired the high canopy and gnarled trunks of trees in the places where the understory had died. It was Dirk who revealed to her that the heart of the forest lay under the insect-rich, fern-filled understory, where roots and fungi extend beneath the loamy soil all the way down to clay, or to the water table.

Now she makes her way through the forest whenever possible to exalt in its lush vitality, observing every detail from the soil underfoot to misty moss-covered bark to the clouds that infuse cedar boughs with moist, oxygen-rich air. She is in heaven here, free from the horrors of the sand line and the nihilism of the streets. She can't wait to talk to Leon, a restoration guilder who is on leave from his post in Haida Gwaii.

When she reaches the first cluster of tree houses, Rafa stops and looks up at the second-growth forest, which is dominated by trunks and treetops that look like giant forearms and hands.

Large heptagonal tree houses rest like bracelets on those arms. On closer observation, she can see that the tree-side walls of the houses are short and windowless. Their roofs extend out and up to cover the outside walls and decks. Below each tree house hang two rope stairways that form a double helix around the supporting trunk. The floors are held up by arrays of slender pilings that penetrate the ground far below. Dangling from the stout branches of nearby trees are hammocks, ropes, bear boxes, and many kinds of storage containers of various sizes.

Rafa spots a man descending a rope and recognizes his long scraggly beard, which she has seen in the dining room at mealtimes. He asks jovially, "Can I help?"

"I'm looking for Leon."

"That's Léon. He's a Francophone from the East Coast."

"Lay-own?"

"Close enough. He appreciates the effort. He's by the third pod, that one up there with the blue roof, probably in his hammock." The man points to a rough, green hammock hidden in the canopy.

"Thanks!"

He darts by and on down the hill. On impulse Rafa asks, "What was your initiation project?"

The man turns and walks nimbly backward downhill. "Shellfish farming."

"Are you glad you did it?"

"Every time I eat shellfish." He turns and runs, and soon disappears into the forest.

Rafa leaves the trail to stand beneath the hammock and call, "Lay-own?"

She hears a groan and a deep growl. "Yes?"

"Would you tell me about your initiation project?"

Fingers poke out between twisted strands of twine. A voice exclaims eagerly, "Rafa! Rafa Aboulafia? Sure! Meet me in the pod." The fingers retract. A shaven head rises above the hammock. Smooth arms reach up and grasp an overhead branch.

Rafa starts up the rope stair, which swings alarmingly. After a difficult climb, she gains the deck and finds Léon, a short animated wraith whose voice betrays no accent. He touches shoulders with Rafa in an intimate greeting that Rafa has seen but not tried before. Behind Léon is a long table flanked by two benches. On the table sits a decanter ringed by glasses. Rafa goes to the deck rail to look down at the forest floor far below, and then to the windows to look inside. She sees nothing but darkness. "This is really something. Will you show me around?"

"Cert." Léon leads Rafa inside, saying in rapid-fire, "This pod is a minimalist one for men who want simplicity and silence—but they're out, so we can talk."

"Were you looking for silence?"

"No!" Léon gestures expansively around the tidy interior. "Six of the seven inner walls have built-in bunks—like that one on the left. That's mine, and so is the counter behind the outer glass. I use it as a desk. The man who lived here before me built shelves and a chair to go under it, and I put a footlocker under the bed. We're standing in the entry—the seventh space—and this is the washroom."

"Can I see it?"

Léon opens the door. The room is a little bigger than the head of Doug's boat, and has an inner window and shower curtain made of tightly-woven fibers. Rafa pushes the curtain aside to find a compact square tub with a low seat, hand-held showerhead, and long lever. "What's that lever?"

"The pump handle. We pump water from the hot springs

into the tub, or—if we want a shower—into the reservoir on the roof. The drain leads down a pipe and on into a sewer that leads to the sea."

"I didn't see a pipe."

"You have to look carefully. It's made of wood—leaks like poison."

"Can't you send the gray water to the garden?"

"We'll get around to it one of these days. Plenty to do. If I had a say, I'd work on the desalination first, bring up enough sea water for our use."

"Does the toilet drain the same way?"

"It's a honey pot. We gather moss and layer it on our night soil. That starts it composting in the can. When it's ready, we send it down and take it to agro."

"Why are you in the silent house?"

"I'm in shakedown. They put me in quarantine."

"What's shakedown?"

"Long story. Let's go out." Léon leads Rafa out through the sliding glass wall to the table and sits in front of the decanter. Sitting opposite, she notices that the central board is recessed on either side of the decanter; in these recesses grow tabletop gardens of tiny plants. She touches a garden's dewdrops and runs her fingers over the contours of its soft green moss.

Léon lifts the decanter. "Forest tea?"

Rafa looks through the golden liquid. "Claro. Can't pass that up."

Léon hands Rafa a half-full glass. She takes a large draft, makes a face, and coughs. Léon laughs. "It's like drinking the temperate rain forest—with a soupçon of sage from the high desert."

"It's like drinking a bog—or eating dirt."

"Thank you. We do that you know—eat soil from the hot houses. In small amounts, it restores the symbionts."

"Restores what?"

"The soil organisms that coat our skin and gut; they join us to our habitat."

Rafa takes a sip of tea, coats her palate, and invites the taste to inform her senses. "I don't get it. Why do you get it? Is it because you're Québecois?"

"I'm Métis—half voyageur and half forest-dweller. I love all soils."

"Why come here?"

"The rainforest. I love the abundant life—I feel good in it."

"Tell me the long story?"

Léon says eagerly, "It started when I fell in love with my initiation project."

"Is that a problem?"

"It can be. It was for me. I lost my grounding in the earth and the body of life." Remembering weakens Léon's focus; he is far away already. His energy body falls into disarray like a stack of satin pillows and slips into the unseen. Even Rafa can feel it.

She feels uneasy. "That must have been some project."

Léon frowns, struggles to regain focus, and continues. "It was. I ran across a patch of wind-felled trees on Van island. It wasn't decomposing. No decomposition, no soil; no soil, no restoration. I decided to try and accelerate the process. It was raining and I was near healthy forest, so I collected fungi and insects and cut them into the dead logs and set them into the ground below. Nothing happened for weeks, so I took it as my project and made it work. The area went from gray, dry, and barren to green, wet, and lush. I couldn't wait to take on a bigger parcel as my vocation project. My consort fell in love with me falling in love with that.

He followed me to help me restore a clear-cut on Haida Gwaii."

"Sounds idyllic. What gave?"

"I got excited—too excited, hyper-focused and monomani-acal. It was tough on my consort. He left. I broke down. I barely got myself home."

"Are you … getting better?"

"I'm on fire to go back, but my energy body is a mess. My counselor put me in quarantine so it wouldn't spread, but his yoga and meditation and energy transfers aren't working. I've learned to focus on my central channel. It helped, but it didn't cure me, and I'm going nuts in the hammock; I'm too isolated. When I do get a chance to talk, I can't stop. I hope you're okay with all of this."

"I'm used to intense hell states; I don't expect a problem. But you were probably wide open and sensitive when you went north."

"The counselor says that I idealized my habitat and my project and took that as my consort. We were simple-same and were living as complex-same—but only in my head. It was a kind of *folie à un*—or *trois*. They don't know. They're afraid of me. That's why they're keeping me at a distance. I don't know how much longer I can do this. When I'm in the hammock, I start pining for my consort and my habitat and my project and I come apart again."

"My dad calls that social deprivation disorder."

"What does he do for it?"

"The opposite of what you're doing. I wonder—*Tío* says—*Tío* thinks there are diseases of every aspect of the body, including interbeing. Maybe you got disconnected from some part of inter-being that was necessary to you."

"*Bien sur.* But what? My counselor says that my grounding in the body of humanity was always weak. He says it's happening more and more as families get smaller and smaller and children have trouble grounding themselves in families and larger aggregate bodies—like communities and habitats. They worry that my problem will spread to the children."

"These children? They get attention and care—and love—from everyone. Your counselor should worry about street kids."

"If I could ground my body in the community and habitat, I could relax into them and they'd mend me."

"They won't let you try?"

"They worry that I'll become an empty with no center, so they delude themselves into thinking they know what to do. Doug says that's the fundamental modern fallacy, and they don't know how to put it behind them."

"Can't you take charge of your own body?"

"Yukie says I should spend time with natural tantrikas. Dirk says you're one; I think so too. I can feel your body grounding mine."

"That's strange. I can't."

"Belatanu's one, too. He learned at an early age to strengthen his energy core, and to use that to stay in sync—to restore life continuously. The rest of us immigrants have gone through processes of loss and gain that join or oppose us to parents or playmates. Those wasted energy and they're hard to get rid of."

"I'm struggling with that. I react to everything the way I react to my father."

"You're a natural. You'll start to sync soon."

Rafa looks at the cedar boughs that shelter the roof and tries to picture her energy body being like its trunk. Something inside her resists. She doesn't want the responsibility. She says uncertainly, "I can't believe that. It would be like getting something for nothing."

Léon grunts. "That's why concepto elders don't talk about naturals. They work really hard for their strength and independence. They don't like to think about children earning time credits so early in life."

"*Tío* has time credits from his work in the Amanas. I feel like I don't have any—or like I spent them on something."

"I'd like to rack up a few by mending my energy body. Dirk says I should consult a warrior elder. He thinks they know the most about the energy body—especially the ones who also belong to concepto, like Wind Carver."

"Why would they know the most?"

"They work with force. Every time they use it they have to erase its traces. That's difficult and subtle work. Very advanced."

"Why don't you consult one, then?"

"I'd have to talk my elders into it first. I don't want any more trouble."

"I'm happy to visit, if that helps. I like it up here, and you're teaching me a lot."

Léon beams. "You're welcome to come when the others are gone—or we could meet in the forest."

Rafa goes to the kitchen next to find the chef, who goes by the name of Cookie. He is darting to and fro between the stove and freezer. Because he is bent forward as he works, his torso whips back and forth. Each time he turns, he sweeps his pitcher ears and pitcher nose back and forth like a coywolf scanning a street for morsels to eat. Rafa wonders how Cookie manages to sync the fast pace of his work with the deliberate pace of his community.

"Cookie?" Rafa calls out tentatively. "Doug said I should ask you about your name." The other agro workers on kitchen rotation stop and stare at her in shock. They pack up their knives, hang their aprons on the hooks by the door, and scurry out. Rafa snorts. "Doug set me up?"

Cookie looks carefully around. Seeing that they are alone, he says, "They all know better than to ask that. But I'll answer your question for Doug's sake. He's the source of all my favorite goodies—cinnamon, chocolate, coffee."

Cookie turns to face Rafa. His face has red-ringed moles and his Adam's apple bulges and moves as he says in a near whisper, "My name is Acre."

"Why not use it?"

"Long story."

"That's probably what Doug wanted me to hear. I'm researching initiation projects to get a better idea of what I should do."

"Hmm. All right. The name is from my first vocation project. I earned my initiation with a project on rapid restoration, and expected to earn my vocation the same way. I found an acre in the Yukon and tried to restore its species balance in three years. When I moved there, I mapped out every living organism, and made it an Eden land. I decided to stay and expand it for my lifework. I took the name Acre to mark my beginning."

"What happened?"

"Lightning struck and burnt it all to the ground."

Rafa opens her mouth to say shit, but the people here use that word as a compliment. She says lamely, "How awful. How did you escape?"

"I waded into the river. Fortunately, no tree fell on me, and rain put out the fire. I asked for a food drop, ordered supplies through Doug, and got ready to start over." Cookie snorts ironically and wipes his hands on his soiled apron. "But winter was coming, and I needed a place to stay, so I took time to build a small cabin on the riverbank. By the time the first snow fell, I had plenty to eat, more than enough to do, and more reason than ever to do it. But I wasn't right. I started to sink."

"Syncing is good, isn't it?"

"I mean my energy—my mood—was falling. I was prepared for darkness and isolation, but not for sterile desolation. I was losing energy. I tried to ramp it up by creating interest and variety. I built a hothouse and planted root vegetables and squash, taught myself to forage for edible mushrooms and herbs, and learned to catch fish and game. I should have been thriving, but I kept losing energy instead of gaining it."

"What did you do?"

"I played. I had a wood stove and some food, so I turned root vegetables into chips, and brined and smoked and pickled fish and game, and made bread and beer, and contemplated nourishment. I filled with energy. My core was like iron. My life changed completely."

"How?"

"My worldview shifted. I saw the fire as an abrupt and frightening way of transferring and transforming nutrients. I saw my body as a furnace that I could stoke with food and use for the dynamic transformation of matter and energy. I wanted to feed the human fire—to restore the human body. So I switched to the hospitality guild and synced—with a y—instead of sinking—with an i. And now I practice a tangible art with tastes and aromas and nutrients that enriches our communion when we break bread together."

"That's hearty and delicate—like a good crust," Rafa says with a smile.

"You got it!" Cookie says with a grin. "Now get out—and look scared!"

Rafa goes next to the dining room. She pauses inside the door to scan the room for a short young woman with smooth bronze skin, broad features, and curly mahogany hair. A girl like that is standing by the sideboard; Rafa has seen her there before. Rafa approaches and flashes a crooked smile that she hopes is disarming. "Are you Kim Coltrane?"

"Why?" she asks absently. Before Rafa can reply, the girl darts gracefully to the corner of the buffet, removes a nearly-empty chafing dish of back bacon, and disappears into the kitchen. A moment later she glides back with a filled dish, returning it to its place and resuming hers. Rafa can't imagine why the girl filled it as much as she did; the dining room is emptying rapidly and she sees few meat-eaters among those who remain. Despite this, as they talk, the dish empties, partly because Rafa helps herself to bacon on toast.

"Doug suggested that I ask you about your initiation project."

Kim continues to regard the room. Rafa is not sure that Kim is listening, until she says, "I'm a performance guilder—a dancer and choreographer. I oversee group movements. During mealtimes, I facilitate the flow of staff and diners."

Rafa's face opens in surprise. "I'm glad I didn't try to guess!"

Rafa stands back by Kim and looks at the dining room. The light spreaders and the ample south and west windows provide bright illumination. The tables are heavy and simple in design and display the close grain of old- or first-growth fir. They have been rubbed with linseed oil until they gleam. Above hang orange paper streamers that signal the approach of harvest.

Kim continues, "Everything tends toward chaos, even move-ment—especially in complex settings like this, where flow is altered by sudden changes like a diner deciding to get syrup, or to talk with a friend sitting beside a busy aisle."

"It doesn't look like a dance."

"I don't choreograph kinesthetic expression or visual display. I coordinate ease and nourishment." Kim smiles. "That was the premise of my project."

"It's like skateboarding in a busy bowl."

"That's jagged. This is refined and restorative—and beautiful when everyone moves as one—it's a form of union."

"Doesn't that happen by itself?"

"It can. Yuko-Hyun has the Japanese skill of choreographing her movements in accord with those of a group. To see what happens without my work, come back when the dining room is packed—say halfway through dinner—and fix your eyes on the wall above the windows. Your peripheral vision will trace our trajectories and reveal their rhythm and patterns. Then move a table or a chair and discover how obstruction causes confusion and deviation—and dissent. I've been watching you and your uncle. You two are dissenters."

"Because we're awkward?"

"Because you inspire change. You create movements that resemble pas de deux, or contrapuntal sequences. You invite us to take new steps. Bloodline advocates like Leilani and Siobhan call themselves dissenters, but they're disrupters. They try to impose fixed or fractious patterns. They interfere with and weaken us."

"Maybe they're here to sharpen your skills, or to challenge you."

Kim smiles knowingly. "You're like your grandmother."

"What makes you say that?"

"I know the performer enacting her. She moves like you do, and says what you would say."

"How could she know about my grandma?"

"From Sarah, Doug, and John. Melissa moved like a dissenter. She went ahead, kept pace, or lagged behind—halted, pivoted, took tangents. And sometimes others followed her."

Rafa feels exposed. She has never considered the responsibility that goes with awareness of movement. She stands as still as a boulder in a valley and watches her thoughts move and collide and scatter.

Kim turns and moves backward, saying, "One moment." She moves gracefully and swiftly toward a staff member who has been standing idle by the drinks buffet, and gestures invitingly toward two empty tables. Her gracious stance is that of valued hostess, not director or player. As Kim glides back to the buffet, the staff member takes a basin to the tables, washes them, and puts up their chairs to make it easier to mop up.

Kim pivots and continues, "I chose this project to reconcile a trauma from my time with the Restorationists."

"Restorationists?"

"They restore habitats, too. They've created a number of Eden lands that have begun to expand without human aid, but they rely on old social patterns. If you want to live in the past, live with them. Every man a tyrant and brute, every woman a slave."

"How can restoration be destructive?" Rafa asks, eyes narrowed. She cannot tell if Doug has sent her to see initiates whose projects were exemplary—or cautionary.

"One moment." Kim crosses the dining room to a group of people who are lost in conversation and blocking the entry. As she guides them graciously to the door, she signals the staff to clear the buffet and dining tables, and beckons Rafa to help clean tables. As they work, Kim replies, "The Restorationists ignore the time debts—the remainders—that they create."

"Like moderns."

Kim pauses to stretch. She twists her ribcage from side to side and tips her chin back. She lifts her head and stands a little taller. "Their leaders cue dominance or submission or exclusion with discordant movements. I did the opposite, and learned to turn discord into dialogue, and dialogue into love."

Rafa raises her eyebrows skeptically. "Can you show me?"

"You've seen it, and I've just explained it," Kim laughs. "You take it for granted. I did too—until I studied the ritual movements of Japanese tea practice, and time and motion studies, and sacred forms of movements like Gurdjieff and Qi Gong. I had already studied ballet and contact improv."

"I'll be watching for what you've told me. Which is good. My perceptions are … under construction."

Next, Rafa lopes down through the forest and out into the clearing. She spots Björn behind the glassblowing oven, carrying a long pole tipped with red-hot glass and wearing a mask. She notes that he has an air of authority; rumor has it that he is a complex-any who has sexually initiated many students. She would like to ask, but she has learned that the topic is taboo. Björn opens the furnace door and plunges the pole into its blazing light. Rafa waits while he pulls it back out, sets it down on a metal frame, and spins it. As he works, he calls out instructions punctuated by belly laughs. Björn's energy is mature, expansive, and grounded. Rafa feels a rush of relief and realizes that she has found what she wants.

Rafa makes a beeline for Björn. "Will you mentor my initiation project?"

Björn's thick brows lift outward like the wings of a bird. "Why not? Should be good for a laugh. What is it?"

"I don't know yet," Rafa confesses.

Björn bellows, "Hey, Mo!"

A svelte young man with disheveled white-blonde hair and deep blue eyes pokes his head through the open wall of the fabro building. "You called?"

"Give me a hand?"

"I was just about to prepare the mold for the panels."

"The fertility center's décor can wait. The dining hall's short on plates."

"Can't have that. Be out in a tick."

Rafa asks, "What was your initiation project?"

"My parents came out to recover from the Great Poisoning, but it was too late. They'd got cancer. I wanted to do something in medicine, but couldn't work it out. I'll show you what I did instead."

Mo lopes to Björn's side and takes his hat, pole, and seat, saying, "We should pour the plates next time. These don't hold up to heavy use."

"That would consume less energy but more material. Let's talk it through. Right now, we need four dinner plates and a dozen glasses."

Mo says, "Right-o."

Björn walks briskly toward the fabro complex.

Rafa runs after him, asking, "So how did you choose your project?"

"I went on walkabout, gave it a think, and decided to have a little fun."

Björn gives Mo a last look and leads Rafa through the open wall of the nearest building. He pauses to shake up the riveting team and to troubleshoot the hoisting of a roof. Everyone who sees him responds like a player eager for improvement. When they reach the other end of the building, Björn enters the long central hallway, and then a door on the right, where he grabs a repurposed ship's wheel that faces a block of storage bins. As the wheel turns, a ponderous end bin rolls outward to open an aisle between it and the second unit. He continues until the aisle has moved far enough to separate the seventh and eighth units.

"You sure you didn't study engineering?" Rafa asks. "A student I knew had shelves like this. Organized. Neat. Complete."

"You don't learn that in school, you learn it in diapers," Björn winks. "All right, then. What's initiation meant to do?"

"Prepare you for independent adult living," Rafa says by rote.

"In your words. Be specific."

"It's a test like any other. You watch, listen and repeat, and tell people what they want to hear until they take you for one of them."

Björn groans. "Initiation is what you make it, mate. Dirk used it to become a man. You don't want to use it to become a tool, do you?"

Rafa squirms inside. "No, but my teachers in Denver—"

"Are far away."

Suddenly, a metal object is hurtling toward Rafa's chest. She moves to catch it. It strikes her middle finger and opens a box of pain. She watches the joint swell. "You sprained my finger!"

"You did that, mate. Listen up! Use your initiation project to become ready for anything and everything. It's like Hamlet says—the readiness is all."

"I don't see how this helps me choose a project."

"Don't search for a perfect project; pick one and use it to become ready to act from your core in good conscience at all times, in the blink of an eye. It's best to have fun because that makes you keen—and open to inspiration."

"Pick a project, any project?" She is peeved, but finds that she cannot remain annoyed with Björn. He radiates fearlessness, and his energy goes right through her as if she weren't there—or were made of air. Rafa looks at the metal object in her hand. "Was this your project?"

"Nope." Björn enters the aisle, reaches into a box, and pulls out a black object. He tosses it into Rafa's ready hands. They shoot upward. Björn smiles.

"Better to overestimate the weight of an object. Now tell me what you see."

Rafa examines it closely. It is a thick-walled cylinder, sleek, smooth, and shiny like lacquerware inside and out. A tap of her fingernail yields a high, dull sound. The sawed-off bottom reveals a cross-section that shows layers of slightly porous, friable material separated by layers of fiber mesh. "A ceramic pipe that preserves heat and conducts electricity?"

"Right in one. Now try and break it."

Rafa drops the cylinder and jumps on it. Nothing happens. "It's strong."

"Strong enough for our purposes."

"But not strong enough to meet engineering standards?" she asks smartly.

"Precisely. I was halfway through my project before I realized it would be foolish to design something for mass production and marketing, or for a special application like space travel. Then I realized that I had no idea how to design something for our needs. So I came up with a few working questions, like what skills and materials do we have in abundance, and how will we stress our pipe, and what earthly forces does it have to withstand. Then

I spent time pondering what pipes could do that they hadn't done before. I decided it would be better to replace pipes than to over-engineer them, so I took the hard decision to ignore the risk of a big earthquake. When I reported all this to Andy, he said I was a fabro designer and asked me to form a new guild."

"Could I create a new vocation?" Rafa asks.

"You don't plan that beforehand; you plan a project and see it through."

"How did you figure all that out with no special training?"

"Experience. I tried to become a performance guilder, but the director always put me on set design and construction. I took the hint and Andy packed me off to Van City to audit a few fabro classes. I went wooly bully for glassmaking and ceramics and came back to apprentice."

"Why did you make the pipe?"

"We ran short on copper, and we needed some for electronics repair. Andy asked me to figure out a way to scavenge and replace the copper pipes. I decided to design a new kind of pipe."

Rafa admires it. "How did you do it?"

"I played in the shop, made half a dozen molds and filled them with mixes of sand, alder sap, pulverized waste glass, and crushed polymer. Then I made that Viking forge and set the molds in it at various distances from the fire, covered them with clay, and let the fire burn. I got lucky. One of the molds at the back made a useable cylinder, and Andy started using the forge to make knives."

"So you had the inner layer. Then what?"

"I glazed and fired it, added a sleeve of glass and iron mesh in concrete for conduction, and also an outer layer of cedar fiber and cob insulation."

"How did you know when it was good enough?"

"Good on ya', mate. That's the hardest step. I wanted to play. I wanted to add an inner layer that cleaned itself. But Andy said, 'You have to know when you're done.' So I stopped."

"Isn't it brittle?"

"Yes. It won't stand up to a serious earthquake."

"What if a kid puts a marble down the drain?"

"They can't do it. Each drain has a cleanable filter and a grate. Nothing passes but liquids and particles."

"Can you show me where you put the pipes in?"

"Nuh. There aren't any. Put one in and had to take it out."

"Oh no! Why?"

"Too much non-ionizing radiation emission. We'd cut way back on electricity, and switched to DC, and we thought we were good there, but luckily Sarah consulted Melissa and found out that we'd be charging the water and metal and spreading and creating dirty electricity. No way to fix it in a retrofit. So I made another sample that was metal-free and we went with that."

"What if I don't get lucky?"

"Ask for help. I'm in touch with fabricators in every experimental community on the Salish Sea—and with all my initiates."

"What's the hardest problem you've had to solve?"

"Learning to say I can't, or I won't. I learned that from the lighting problem. Our biggest transition after modernity was finding ways to use less power. We used to use heaps, especially in the dark months from November to February. I kept struggling to produce more and more energy and then I realized that I wasn't adapting—or innovating. We had to change our habits first. So I went to Andy and suggested that we adapt to the dark by doing fertility practices in the winter and restoration in the summer. He persuaded the founders to lead that change. Now the theater is our biggest energy spender, which is the reason we went for the stationary cycle block behind the low earthen wall."

Rafa looks around furtively and lowers her voice. "Someone implied that I'd be taking sexual initiation. Am I supposed to include that in my project?"

Rafa can feel Björn laughing behind his blank expression. "No, sweet pea. We go through a full course in the fertility center that takes care of all of that. You can't do that in time for the legacy enactments, so Sarah decided to count them as your initiation. But if I were you, I'd go over there, sit in on some classes, and request a practical initiation."

"You mean physical union?"

"Right-o."

"I do have experience. And I don't want to have sex with a teacher."

"Look, mate, it's our specialty. You may as well take advantage."

"What did you declare?"

"I'm a solitary. My initiation was forty-eight hours of ecstasy—after which I was two days farther from finding a life partner and sharing meaning and purpose. So I opted out. For now."

"What should I do first—for the fabro project?"

"Come back tomorrow and I'll put you on each of the teams, give you a chance to develop some skills. And then you'll propose a project."

Rafa laughs. "Where do you want me to start?"

"Why don't you let Mo start you on glass? You'll learn to pay attention—or get a burn you won't forget."

"Tomorrow? That'll work."

Newly energized, Rafa soon bounds up to the bucolic agro center, which reminds her of the children's petting zoo at the

Denver stock show. She pauses to admire the small hand-cropped pasture and to inhale the low notes of compost-rich soil and the top notes of sweet grass. She spots Dirk's friend Belatanu pushing a wheelbarrow filled with manure toward the massive compost heap in the clearing beyond the west fence. He is wearing a deer-skin hat that hides his large features, and a short coverall that reveals his imposing physique as well as a geometric tattoo that extends from his bronzed nape down to his wrists and knees.

Rafa rushes to catch up. "Hey, Bel! Tell me about your initiation project?"

"Why? You want to do the same one?" Belatanu teases good-naturedly. His calm, kind grounding anchors Rafa and frees her playfulness.

"Not after Björn's lecture on how it has to come from my core."

"I've heard that one." Belatanu laughs. "Help me with this, and I'll help you."

Rafa grabs the wheelbarrow. "Can you feed everyone with this tiny farm?"

"If the guests don't eat too much."

Rafa laughs and nearly tips the barrow.

Belatanu opens the west gate, removes his hat, and runs a hand over his coarse black hair. Rafa pushes the barrow through and sets it down at the edge of the compost pile. She pulls a pitchfork from her side of the pile; Belatanu grabs his own from the other. They heft clods of manure onto the pile and mix it in. The work is heavier than she expected. She has to use her foot to push the fork into the pile, and works up a sweat.

Belatanu pauses to say, "You should go for agro. Manure is for sure."

"You've just talked me out of it." Rafa grins.

They resume their work. When they finish, they cover the pile with cut grass and push the pitchforks into it. Then he pushes the barrow back through the gate and heads for the barn. Rafa says, "I do like animals. I miss dogs."

"At least they don't get up to crazy schemes like legacies."

"What's wrong with legacies?"

"I question Sarah's ambition. We've done enough for the biosphere. We could use some ease and renewal."

"Goddard! Over here!" shouts a voice from the barn. Rafa turns to see a woman in a deerskin hat and leather boots.

"Did she just call you Goddard?"

"She called me goat herd. That's what they call the person on goat duty."

Ten minutes later, Rafa is in the goat shed milking a tiny white goat with straw-colored horns. "So what was your project?"

"Take a look at the feed."

Rafa looks over her goat's back at the trough from which she is eating. "It's green and red!"

"We used to cultivate all our feed. I was the one who introduced foraging. It started when Dirk and I were down at the beach skipping stones at low tide. We walked over a dozen lines of smelly dead seaweed washed up on shore. I noticed sea lettuce tossing in the waves in front of us and had an epiphany. We could eat it, and the animals could eat it. We'd been taught not to eat anything in the sea because of the red tide, but I knew I had to figure it out, so I made it my project."

"So all you had to do was figure out when to harvest it?"

Belatanu laughs. "And what kind to harvest, and where, and how to preserve it, and what various animals would eat, and how it affected their milk and cheese, and so on and so on."

"You did all that for one project?"

"No. The trick for that was to define the first step. I figured out how to harvest and preserve red sea lettuce, made up some mixes to try, figured out what Sadie here would eat, and also what effect it would have on her cheese. It was a big project, but fun and profitable. Her cheese has a special flavor—it tastes like chalk to me, but some food lovers in town can't get enough of it. Their dinner club provides our olive oil in exchange for all her cheese. She's as valuable as our cranberry bog."

"Dirk says you linked initiation and vocation. I'd like to do that."

"I chose vocation first—well, it chose me. When I was in school, and Parvati had just started teaching, she had us hatch a clutch of duck eggs. She didn't tell us about imprinting—she wanted us to figure it out. I was amazed and thrilled when they hatched and started following me everywhere. They didn't follow anyone else. The same thing happened the next year when we hatched chicks, and again when we rescued a baby ouzel. Later, I found out I could step right into the salmon spawning area without getting attacked. So I accepted that agro had chosen me."

"Aaron said that in the Amanas they use animals to choose medicos."

"Oh, no! I should have been a doctor!"

"Or a body worker or a counselor."

"The animals do like my touch. But they don't say much."

Rafa laughs and says, "Can I ask you a personal question?"

"I thought you'd been doing that."

Rafa smiles. "Are you Salish?"

"Samoan."

"What's that?"

"Samoa's an island in the Pacific. My mother's people lived in Polynesia until the water level rose and flooded them out."

"Well, skunk me. I thought you must have had it easy, but you only make it look that way. No wonder you want ease and renewal."

Belatanu stands, pats Sadie on the rump, and picks up the milk bucket. "Do us a favor and persuade Sarah we can't do everything."

"I doubt she'll listen. *Tío* says she's been planning his legacy project for years. Another personal question?"

"That'll cost you another milking."

"No time."

"Make it quick, then."

Rafa notices that Beltanu's state feels different than Björn's; it's grounded, transparent, intense, and strongly masculine, but also peaceful and somehow bottomless. "I heard Parvati's a celibate—that a lot of you are. Are you?"

"No. I'm a simple-diff, looking for a first consort."

"Really? But you're so ... " Rafa blushes. She wants to hold him. The urge is strong, and she does not particularly want to resist it. "Do you date first? Or, um, practice union?" Suddenly she feels exposed, and brazen. And anxious. She does not want to spoil their budding friendship, but friendship is not what she wants. Perhaps it's all this talk of sexuality and fertility. Whatever the reason, she's falling for him fast.

"We get to know each other," he says, with an expression she can't read. "And then we commit for a year. That way we can explore our shared fertility, see if we discover a third."

"And if you don't?"

"Depends. Most move on, some give it more time." He looks at her with an almost stern expression. "Look, if you don't grow up here, and you don't already have a partner, it can be hard to ground yourself here—socially and energetically. Take extra care to keep your energy centered and low. I'd hate to see you go into shakedown."

Rafa follows Belatanu into a room on the other side of the barn, where he pours the milk into a large pan warming on the stove and says, "You know, I'm thinking that if you chose agro, you could have a puppy. We breed working farm dogs, and have three left from the last litter."

"Unfair, my friend. I'd better clear out. Thanks for the advice, Goddard."

"Blissings, Rafa. Don't be a stranger."

Seeing that it is nearly time for lunch, Rafa goes to find Yukie at the schoolhouse. Rafa is relieved to talk to someone from a far-away place who knows what it is like to make this place her home. Yukie gives Rafa a hug and then takes her out to play on the ropes course. Yukie begins, and has such fun and such a beautiful ability to share it that Rafa spends a good five minutes on the ropes before asking for the tour of the inside of the school that they had skipped when the bear bell rang.

Yukie, who is falling into the role of big sister, takes Rafa inside, where she sees arrays of cubbyholes and cabinets covering the wall on either side of the door. In them are shoes; yoga mats; personal futons; clay for sculpting; twine for weaving; paints; and performance aids like masks, flutes, and bark robes. She follows Yukie to the opposite wall and helps pull out wheeled, fern-topped shelf units, arranging and equipping them to form a library and a biochemistry laboratory. Yukie measures the humidity and sets out a decorative basket of dried mosses to regulate the air.

Rafa exclaims, "This is amazing! How did you get all these ideas?"

"For my project, I researched traditional Japanese and Korean designs and the Living Building paradigm that the founders adopted and developed. So some of the ideas are ancient—like the futon cupboards and tatami mats for the little ones' naps—and some are recent, like the moveable walls and bio-filtration of indoor air."

"It seems like everything is alive—or was," Rafa says, plopping down on a stray cushion. "This is comfy! What's in it?"

"Shredded cedar bark. Björn taught me how to harvest it. I designed the east wall myself." Yukie leads Rafa to the east wall, which is made of very thick reed paper that takes water stylus images which evaporate on their own. She picks up a stylus and draws a leaf, and then tries several more of varying widths. They do not evaporate. "Why isn't it working?"

"It takes a light touch and a few minutes—which has the added benefit of making you think about what's most important to write."

Lastly, they admire the objects suspended from the ceiling grid—the antique lighting instruments for student projections as well as audio/visual players, microphones, and speakers. Rafa is used to technology but also wary of it, yet here she finds she trusts it. Still, she prefers the models, artifacts, and artworks that the students made by hand, which are on display on the high shelves under the grid.

"This is like a one-room schoolhouse with ten rooms!"

"It's very space efficient, which is energy efficient and also keeps us outside and active and healthy."

Rafa pulls out a futon and a tatami mat and lays down on them. The futon is for under-sevens, so her legs stick out comically. Yukie does the same, and they stare at the ceiling for a minute. She breaks the silence by describing the exterior, which was more difficult for her to design, and which she hopes will be redesigned. She points out the south half of the roof, which is made of glass, and the north half, which is covered with sod and edible, fragrant herbs. Those Rafa likes, but the cedar, moss-lined walls are waterproofed with bear grease that has a bad smell, and the moss is either dry and poorly insulating, or wet and rotting the cedar.

"I want to try one," Rafa says. "Maybe a newer version of the clinic Melissa designed. *Tío* was telling me that it worked well but biodegraded a bit too fast." Relaxed by the intimate feel of lying side by side on futons, she asks, "What is it that everyone sees in Dirk?"

"You don't see it?"

"I like him. He's interesting. But I don't 'like' like him."

"He has the kind of energy we all want to have. We work hard at it, but he could do it before he could walk. I guess you have to have been here a while to get it."

"I guess so."

"Must be nice for him that you don't want him. Everybody else wants something from him. And I mean everybody."

"What did he declare?"

"Sarah didn't let him. She's sending him out to a post in the north to live on his own for a year or so. She says if he doesn't get time away, he'll never know his true inclinations."

"Is that what people mean by empty?"

"An empty is someone with no core who doesn't add to the community. Like a parasite. It's insidious."

"Isn't that shakedown?"

"Shakedown is probably a problem with interbeing, but they don't really know."

"What do you think of Belatanu?"

"He's a friend. Why?"

"I think I like him as a man. I just want to jump him!"

"Really? That's great for him."

"Why?"

"We tend to feel him as sad."

"Really? To me he's really serene. And grounded—like a tree."

"I get that. He does keep his energy low and strongly centered, and you—you feel like you might fly away on your enthusiasm. Personally, I love it; we could use more of that. But that's because I'm better grounded than most."

"Maybe that's why I feel good around you. But don't worry. I don't find you any sexier than Dirk."

"I'll take that as a kudo."

12

Intruders

That evening, after dinner, Rafa looks for Sarah to ask her advice about a project that might create a new guild for fabro trading. After looking for some time, she finds Kim, who points Rafa to Sarah's room. Rafa listens keenly at the closed door to make sure she isn't disturbing anything before knocking softly. After a long pause, Parvati opens the door and draws Rafa into the room. Sarah is sprawled on the bed in her white robes, cane hooked on the head of the bed. Yuko-Hyun is rummaging through the armoire. Rafa looks around the tiny room. In addition to the usual bed and desk and armoire, it holds several works of art and a row of straight-backed twig chairs that stand beneath a bark board dotted with vintage photos, some of which include her grandmother.

Yukie pulls Sarah's nightclothes from the armoire, closes it, and sits next to Sarah on the bed. As Yukie gently lifts Sarah's head onto her pillows, Rafa sees with a shock that Sarah is exhausted and irritable. Rafa has never seen her like this. She feels a stab of anxiety; she has seen Sarah as the mother who keeps things running in the background, holding them all above the mire of indecision, uncertainty, and ultimate responsibility. She does not want to think that Sarah or Doug could fail the whole community. The specter of mortality that Rafa evaded by plunging freely into sanguine expectations and adventure now returns to laugh and point at her, trapping her on a social island within a bigger social island where the weight of decisions that affect all their safety, wellbeing, and freedom may fall on her.

Parvati leads Rafa to the twig chair closest to Sarah, and gestures for Rafa to sit down.

Sarah frowns and says sharply, "Well?"

"I'd like some advice."

Sarah attempts to recover her composure. She takes a deep breath and says decidedly, "I'm going to need more help. Yukie, go and bring back a few of the fertility guilders from our support team."

Yuko-Hyun bows and darts out of the room. Parvati sits beside Sarah. Rafa feels the room fill with gentle love that reminds her of her mother and puts her at ease. Within the minute, her heart lifts and fills her field of vision with white light that shimmers and turns blue.

They hear another knock. Rafa jumps up to open the door, and finds Dirk standing in the corridor with an unfamiliar warrior. Rafa nods and takes her seat as the two men enter the tiny space. The unfamiliar warrior crouches beside the foot of Sarah's bed like a runner in the starting blocks. Sarah adjusts her position with effort and asks with forced calm, "Yes?"

"A cluster of six fear addicts in polar military surplus gear is coming south toward the memorial. They have with them murder weapons from several eras—including old ordnance."

Sarah looks stunned. She asks the warrior to repeat himself. When he finishes, she looks at Parvati in astonishment and then clarifies, "South? They're coming up over the hill with heavy artillery?"

The warrior nods. Rafa feels laughter bubble up behind the warrior's fierce expression and lift their spirits in the face of this urgent and troubling news.

"Some time debts are too, too tenacious!" Sarah exclaims, exasperated. "We'll never be done with the consequences of militarism! Fear, fear, fear, fear, fear, and pretty soon—murder!" She takes another deep breath, grasps Parvati's hand, and says formally, "The intruders' actions speak for themselves. What do you propose?"

The warrior replies without looking up. "They may know of the net; it's too late to dig a pit, and a fall could harm them. A consort pair is working in the retreat cabin and we don't want the intruders to move in their direction. It will be safest to gather everyone else in the safe room while we climb nearby trees and tranq the intruders."

"You calculated and verified the human dose?"

"We have the right darts at the ready."

"When you have taken them, what will you do?"

"We will take their materials to fabro, take them to a boat in Fulford Harbor, and tow them into the Strait. We'll leave them with the usual supplies and offer of training."

"Good. Proceed. Our good wishes go with you. Godspeed."

The warrior leaps to his feet and runs out, leaving the door open. His footsteps quickly recede down the corridor and the stairs.

"Dirk! Organize lights off and gather everyone in the hot room—what do you call it—the one that blocks infrared sensors."

"Your wish is my command," he teases. He winks and runs out.

Sarah sighs, "Oooof!" She laughs darkly and adds, "I wish we could keep him! I'd love him to stay and share his courage—especially with those of us whose bodies are failing!"

Yuko-Hyun enters with several fertility guilders in yellow

robes. Sarah announces, "We have intruders. Yukie—please gather the rest of the team and go to the hot room for a lights off—and block mine on your way out."

Yukie bows. The fertility guilders fan out around the bed as Yukie goes to turn off the switch behind Sarah's bed and gathers a handful of thick disks from the armoire. She places them around the room. When Rafa's eyes adjust, she sees that the disks are emitting green pinpoints of light, and that Yukie has gone.

Sarah turns to Rafa and says, "Before you go—"

They hear a syncopated rapping at the door. Sarah calls, "Come in, Oke Ten!"

Oke Ten enters and, with difficulty, takes the ritual position of a warrior. "A group of hate addicts is coming and will arrive in several days. Rumors about Aaron and Rafa are triggering fear groups and hate groups. The latter are allied with neighbors who are averse to our ways. "

Parvati gasps in astonishment and asks, "Might our mourning for Melissa be drawing their anger?"

"It could aggravate our neighbors," Sarah says with a low laugh, apparently refreshed by the fertility guilders. "Our species is still avoiding and fighting its grief work, and sorrows can fuel fear and anger, especially in all-male groups."

"How very modern to respond with problems instead of solutions," observes a fertility guilder in a tone of easy wonder that draws Rafa's focus back from the brink of old traps like responding to fear and anger with more fear and anger.

"Please, take a seat, my friend," Sarah says, breaking their formality.

Oke Ten, who rises with difficulty, takes a twig chair, and places it beside Rafa, and then sits down and relaxes. His face falls, revealing his cares and his age. Seeing Oke Ten like this reminds Rafa that it will not be long before the welfare of all who abide in this place will depend on her generation.

Oke Ten asks kindly, "How is the pain in your back?"

Sarah looks for a moment as if she may cry, and then says resignedly, "Time was when I could transform all of the pain in real time, but I'm falling behind more and more, and it's getting the better of me."

"I'm sorry to hear it."

"How's your knee?"

Oke Ten examines it and shrugs. "I tape it." He adds thoughtfully, "We are fortunate that Doug is looking out for us. He warned us of the plot."

Sarah says matter-of-factly, "Please express gratitude to him, and think about what we will do when he is gone." Rafa's courage rises. Her heart commits to her vocation. It has made her decision: she will take Doug as her main mentor, and Björn, too, if she is allowed to make a clinic to sell. She feels suddenly very grown up. They are including her in their ways of governance. They are treating her like a member of the guild and the community, which means that they trust enough in her maturity and ethics to reveal what they do without worrying that she will interfere, take advantage, or spoil their plans.

Sarah says, "Let's take a moment now to pray in silence for Rafa to find her vocation; for the ancient trees that the fear addicts may sacrifice to the old gods of tribalism, fear and attack; and for Oke Ten and the community as we all face new malice."

"And for habitats that depend on our species," Parvati says.

Rafa watches the fertility guilders. As each begins to pray in a different way, their faces become radiant, and she feels their loving kindness and compassion fill the room. After a delicious, restorative minute of silence, Sarah continues.

"Let's see if we can devise a way to undo the plot. Oke Ten, please tell us the whole story."

Oke Ten says, "A network of hate addicts that trades in the barrens found out about us and—"

"How?" Sarah interrupts.

Oke Ten looks at Rafa sadly and says, "A hate addict overheard Aaron speak of us in Missouria. That addict sold the story to a trader. That trader took it to a dominator in Chicago. He alerted malefactors in the Great Lakes slave trade. The story they received was costly and—unfortunately—accurate."

"Do they mean to steal our children?"

"They intend to steal as many of us as they can and sell the fastest among us to sport hunters, the strongest to slavers, and the rest to sex slavers and cannibals."

Rafa can hardly believe what she is hearing. She had felt safe from the evils that nearly destroyed her life back in Denver.

Sarah asks evenly, "When will they arrive?"

"Seventy-two hours, give or take."

"What do you propose?" Sarah asks.

"They will arrive in a sloop. We can take it from below and tow it to Limbo."

"Will other malefactors follow?"

"We don't know. We have been working with other communities to develop a new monitoring system for malefactors. Doug advised this. We alerted the communicator on Quadra, and she is exploring the comm networks for clues."

"Are you coding the messages?"

"Yes, and we communicate in a dialect of Coastal Salish."

"Good," Sarah says decisively. "Let's meet tomorrow morning at eight in the breakfast room to discuss our response and adaptation. Bring three warriors, Oke, and I will bring three elders."

"Will you bring Aaron?" Oke Ten asks.

Sarah smiles. "I'll bring three elders and Doug, and Aaron if he's free."

"Can I join you?" asks Rafa.

"Yes."

"What will happen to the people you tow away?" Rafa asks.

Sarah replies sadly, "We offer to cure them of their habits of hate."

Parvati adds, "We tow any true malefactors to a deserted island in the Bering Strait that we call Limbo. On the way, warriors who have been soldiers share their experiences of transformation. When the boat arrives, the warriors leave supplies and a communicatons device. But so far, they have all returned to Neanderthal ways."

"What do you mean?"

"The most murderous kill the others until there is only one. Sometimes they eat the flesh. The lone survivor may plant a garden and catch fish, but when new malefactors arrive, the killing begins all over again until only one survives."

"Can't the fertility guild restore them?"

"A guilder once tried, but the lone survivor eventually killed and ate her."

"Can't you make peace with them?" Rafa asks with a sick feeling.

"Occasionally, we detect one who has been labeled a malefactor but is still able to exit hell states. We offer her or him the chance to restore a remote habitat. Several have taken up the offer and learned transformation, and two have come to live here at the center."

Rafa feels strangely comforted by Parvati's crisp descriptions of grisly events. Now that Rafa is becoming more aware of states, and learning to turn hellish ones into heavenly ones, she sometimes veers from one kind to the other, but only when she is alone. Now she is calm enough to notice a risk that no one has mentioned.

Rafa says, "Given all of that *Tio* should have a look at the communicator you intend to leave with them on Limbo."

Sarah looks at Oke Ten and says, "I'll bring Aaron in the morning. Rafa, can you let him know?"

"I will."

Oke Ten rises. He takes Sarah's hand in friendship and then resumes his formal warrior bearing, nods to the others, and leaves.

Sarah looks after him and says admiringly, "Not a wasted moment, nor movement—and never any hurry!"

Parvati stands. The women look at Rafa. Sarah asks, "What did you want to ask?"

"You answered it. Thanks." Rafa stands and gives Sarah a kiss on the cheek.

13

Cascadia

S arah stands on the edge of the inner harbor of Victoria watching Gina and her wives walk toward the city center. Above, Devonshire cream clouds sail past on a sea of salty air. Gina's red wavy hair, Lisa's black kinky hair, and Lena's straight blond hair show that they are not blood sisters, but the way that they move and speak and teach as if they were one body and being sometimes prompts Sarah to see their marriage as incestuous.

Sarah turns to the trader's dock in the harbor and to Doug's boat docked in one of the empty slips. As a founding member of their guild, he is guaranteed a mooring; now he is also welcomed as a mentor. Trade is down. Many communities are choosing self-sufficiency and dropping out of the credits system. This short-sighted, self-oriented solution may make it difficult to sustain the best gifts of modernity, the ones the elders are keen to keep, like medicines, helicopter ambulances, and foods that save lives and habitats.

She and Doug do not want to talk about that now. None of the group can do anything about it—except Doug, who has come to boost morale by spending credits and engaging curiosity, and Sarah, who has come to provide a neighboring community with the tough love of mediation that may push them into developing a successful economy.

Aaron and Parvati help Doug keep his balance as he disembarks. Rafa and Belatanu pull up and stow the booster steps and jump down after them. John and Yuko-Hyun and Sarah's support team of three fertility guilders are already on their way up the stairs to the promenade level. Sarah awaits their arrival with gratitude and hope. She has never been this weak, but may yet be able to meet all of her responsibilities with the aid of her trio, each of whom has a special talent for creating and sharing strong states.

Soon they have all ascended and gather in a knot to look up the flax field south of the harbor to the grand old edifice that dominates it. Sarah tells Rafa that the edifice was built to house the Parliament of the old province of British Columbia and has since become the New Guildhall of Cascadia. The office buildings behind it house shared ventures like the Arbitration Centre.

Rafa says, "It looks like the old state capitol in Denver but bigger—and golder."

Doug says, "The gold is from the solar-geothermal exchange panels—they're plain glass and filled with apple brandy."

Rafa laughs. "Why apple brandy?"

"There are plenty of apples, and fermentation produces alcohol that retards freezing and spoilage."

Dora, the tallest and oldest of the fertility guilders, adds in a bubbly voice, "I love the color, and the way the panels appropriate the forest. They extend way down into the ground like roots." Dora puts her arms up in imitation of a tree. Her rough, grayish skin and greenish updo make the imitation uncannily convincing.

Sarah stretches her arms and sighs contentedly. "I never tire of the beauty of this harbor!"

"Really?" Rafa asks incredulously. "I see the end of a voracious empire!"

Ella, the shortest fertility guilder, says, "I do too! I see tons of metal and other materials we can't put back."

Sarah feels Ella's energy contract around her pale, pear-shaped body, and resolves to keep the mood as celebratory as possible.

Selah, the gentlest of the fertility guiders, says, "I see a monument to The War on Life."

Sarah is relieved to feel Selah's equanimity deepen to compensate for Ella's lapse.

John chimes in mildly with, "I see evidence that we're only just beginning to change."

Sarah says, "I see a cautionary history of our species. We refused to choose life until the last minute—until the conventional agricultural lands of California were all poison barrens and sand dunes." All eyes follow Sarah's and fix on Aaron as she asks, "And what do you see?"

Aaron ponders a moment. "That we can and will do better. The ideas behind this type of land use were short-sighted and naive, but the skills that realized them were many and marvelous—and still available to us."

Sarah smiles smugly at Doug, who has been trying to lower Sarah's expectations of Aaron. Doug deflects attention by pointing out the varieties of moss and salal that line the crisscrossed paths, then takes his leave, saying, "We will see you later."

Sarah and her support team sweep Aaron up the New Guildhall path. When they reach the east side of the hall, she turns toward the main doors, saying "Let's go through the hall to the Arbitration Center."

"I'd like that. I remember it from when it was still the Provincial Capitol of B.C."

When they enter, Aaron stops and stares in disbelief. While the outside is barely altered; the interior is unrecognizable. "Good heavens!"

Sarah explains, "As the Provincial government shrank, Victoria became a major hub in Cascadia, and the Capitol Regional District took the initiative in transportation, communications, and trade. In 2030, they invited communities in each of the major and minor watersheds in the bioregion to participate in a transitional bioregional assembly."

"I remember. Mom called it the Althing—after a Viking gathering."

"It was a terrible time. The chemical industry had collapsed and taken others with it—including the industrial agriculture that caused obesity, malnutrition, poisoning, and food allergies, and also the health industry that fed on those problems. Everyone knew modernity was done but few were ready to move on, and most thought it was too late. Halfway through the meeting, I realized that at least a third of the participants were suicidal and might end their lives if the meeting failed."

"It went well in the end."

"After it had come too close to the unthinkable. Had we failed and let each fend for herself, the biosphere would have collapsed with the economy."

"I'm glad the assembly gutted the building instead of each other," Aaron says wryly.

Sarah smiles. "They gutted it and braced the shell with a light grid of carbon steel, then dug down three levels to put in a utility center with a geothermal installation that draws heat from the inner harbor; a black water unit that drains under the front field; an emergency depot for earthquake and tsunami relief; a desalinator with a cistern; a chemistry lab; a comm center—all kinds of shared resources."

"I see the outer wall, the grid, and ... what looks like walls of glass bricks."

"They hold water and act as a thermal mass, and they're etched with abstract views of Cascadia—aerial maps of watersheds and habitats joined by symbols of interweaving like bridges and ships."

"They're stunning—especially with the living ferns and mosses worked in as a hanging garden on a transparent net."

"Behind the hard thermal wall is a soft wall of fiber sleeves with braided comm wires, sensors, switches, pipes, radiation shields, and I don't know what."

"What are those ... towers?" Aaron asks, pointing to the array of nine three-level structures of iron lace that fill the interior below and around the dome, and that are joined by catwalks and staircases with outside box lifts. "They look like unfinished Eiffel Towers."

"Each floor of eight of the towers housed one founding guild. The other is for the guild of the whole—and all guilds outside the original twenty-one."

Aaron hears a shrill scream followed by laughter, and sees three small boys emerge from a tube into a lap pool below the dome. "Is that—a water slide?"

"It's a series of slides for water therapy—and for fun! They're part of the central spa. Guild members can use the pools for relaxation and the dance station for stimulation—it helps them get into optimal states for negotiation or mediation. They can also bring and share any children they have, inspiring us to have fun and look to the future."

Aaron laughs. "It's delightful! There's no place like this in the Amanas. We're subdued, industrious, and loving—but not prone to play or whimsy."

"We—including you—need a place to congregate and connect now that scavengers have disassembled the cities. Thank heaven! Forest dwellers can become isolated—or go feral!"

"I'll bet they don't need arbitration."

Sarah laughs. "Not often. Which reminds me, I need a chair massage to get my body into a fertile state—and one for each of you to get you into care states!"

Twenty minutes later, they exit the Guildhall refreshed. Aaron follows Sarah and her support team into the nearest building behind the hall; they go up its broad, worn stairs to the second floor, where they search the corridor until they find a closed door with a sign reading: "Saturna Saltspring Fishing Rights Dispute."

Sarah opens the door to reveal a room with a scuffed, graying interior of wood planks treated long ago with linseed oil. On their left is a rectangular wooden table at which four people are sitting facing irregular rows of empty chairs. Sarah takes a seat opposite them at the table, while Aaron takes a seat behind her in the front row of the gallery. Dora, Ella, and Selah sit beside him. A man enters and sits beside Sarah; he looks young and fit and desperate. No other members of the public enter to view the open mediation.

Aaron studies the panel of four. On his left is a sour-looking woman with short, high, white hair and wrinkle lines radiating from her features. Beside her is a man in a visor cap who is tall and nearly emaciated. Next to him sits a sad looking man with a sagging face that reminds Aaron of a beagle. On the right sits a tiny woman with protuberant eyes who quivers like a bird.

The sour woman shakes a rattle, and the beagle-faced man asks morosely, "What is Saltspring prepared to offer to cover our costs?"

"What are the costs?" Sarah prompts.

"Twenty credits per side," the sad man replies.

"What is Saturna offering?" she asks.

"Fish," answers the young man.

"Our fish? That is unacceptable to us. We offer five place settings of fine pottery for sale in the market," Sarah counters.

"What does Saturna offer?" asks the beagle-faced man.

"We offer fifty cob bricks for sale in the market."

"Accepted," says the sour woman. "We expect you to deliver those to room one by seventeen hundred hours. Saturna, state your business."

"Twenty years ago," the young man tells the panel of mediators, "you assigned us a three-week fishing season. It has never been enough to feed our families with the boats and crews that we have, so we increased to five weeks this past season and told Saltspring. We gave them fair warning. But when we went out, they sent their warriors to pull our boats back to port! We charge them with stealing our fish and assaulting our boats."

The sour-faced woman nods to Sarah, who says, "You were fishing during our weeks. You were stealing our fish. There can be no crime when we peaceably prevented a crime—and did no harm to person or property."

"You used force! We didn't consent. You have other sources of food, but you took ours. Soon you'll take our land and turn it into a forest!"

"We'd all like to get by on fish, but there aren't enough to go around. That's why we negotiate fishing rights, and that's why we enforce them."

"You have meat and dairy and all kinds of crops."

"We choose to spend our time and resources on agriculture so that we can eat well without depleting wild populations of fish. Instead of doing the same, you take advantage of our commitment and our responsibility."

"We don't have the economy you have."

"Our economy didn't happen to us. We built it, and we continue to build it. We do well because we work hard and well for the good of all."

"You have an unfair advantage—that teaching center. We can't compete."

"There's no competition. You don't face and solve your problems. You want us to do it for you without offering anything in return."

Aaron is beginning to realize that by immersing himself in daily and periodic events, he is beginning to see how much Sarah does inside and outside the Center, how casual her governance— or service—is, and how well it works no matter the circumstances. To be on sounder footing, he will have to probe the history and networks of the community, and ask others for their stories of its genesis, its disasters, and its dreams.

The sour woman shakes a ceremonial rattle. The beagle-faced man declares, "Enough! What do you propose, Saturna?"

"We propose increasing our fishing season to five weeks."

"What is your counter-proposal, Saltspring?"

"If Saturna increases its fishing season, we will withdraw from the fishing agreements and rely on our shellfish farms, which are now productive enough to substitute for wild-caught fish. We will also withdraw the warriors who protect Saturna's fishing rights."

The young Saturna representative sputters, "You—you—you—you're a big island oppressing a little one! You're forcing us to do what you want!"

"On the contrary. You'll be able to do whatever you want—except take advantage of our labor."

As the difference in their positions becomes clearer to Aaron, he feels glad to be part of a community that is large, grounded, competent, and ingenious. They are willing and able to survive—and determined to do so. He can see that some people cling to modernity for fear of the long, slow, desperate failure that comes of being almost resourceful enough to survive—but not quite. He is relieved when Saturna persuades Sarah to send a team of one shellfish farmer, three agro guilders, and two dairy cattle to help them develop new food sources. That resolves the dispute to the satisfaction of all—for now.

As Sarah, Aaron, and the trio who are sustaining angelic states in Sarah's support move quickly up the field toward the former Capitol building, Doug dallies, leading his group at a slower pace. He takes time to build up John and Belatanu's interests in the weekly tournament at the hockey rink that he would like to visit after picking up his special delivery at the traders' center in the great hall. When he reveals this plan, Rafa asks what he is picking up; Doug only smiles slyly and shrugs.

Parvati says, "He's still the boy in the dorm who knows how to be the center of attention!"

Doug teases her back. "You'll never get me to tell you that way!"

Soon, in spite of—or perhaps because of—Parvati's observation, they are all guessing at the nature of the special delivery, and Doug is finding out what each of them wants most—or least. Belatanu does not like things; John likes instruments; Parvati likes ornaments; Yuki likes books about faraway places; and Rafa wants a doctor, body worker, counselor, and habitat restorer trained by her grandmother to staff her clinic.

"You don't ask for much, do you?" Doug says ironically to Rafa. "Don't you need the clinic building first?"

"They'll have a lot to learn when they get here."

"True."

The group enters the Guild Hall, where they go to the first floor of the farthest tower. Like several in other towers, this floor has rooms for meetings; unlike them, this one has an open bar with refreshments and snacks. Doug stops at the entry workstation to sign in on the board and then leads them to the bar, where they all try the effervescent iced cider special from the Okanagon. Doug soon disappears through a door that opens behind the bar, and is screened by lush plants. The group waits and samples the luxuries available, luxuries that those outside the enclosure can see but not taste: olives and pistachios from the south, smoked fish from the north, oysters from the west, and sugar maple syrup from the east.

Sarah, Aaron, and the Trio soon return, find their friends, and try the delicacies advised by the bartender. Then Sarah takes the whole group—minus Doug—on a tour. When they return to the trader's center, they begin to speculate as to what Doug is doing, and then to consider enjoying the water slides while he is occupied. Just as they are about to leave, however, they hear a door open, and see Doug come walking toward them, followed by a small figure cloaked and hooded in burlap. Rafa does not dare to hope or to speculate. She holds her breath.

When Doug reaches them, he steps aside saying, "Here we are."

The figure throws back the hood and smiles broadly, eyes searching. To Doug's surprise and consternation, Rafa bursts into tears and nearly trips as she runs at Mitzi and gives her friend a bearhug; she cannot help it. Mitzi, too, begins to sob, and Parvati, Yuki, and Belatanu shed sympathetic tears even as Parvati asks Doug in bewilderment, "Who have you brought to us?"

"Mitzi, long lost friend of Rafaela from Denver. They left in a hurry, didn't expect to meet again."

Rafa says to Mitzi, between intakes of breath, "You're ... the ... only ... one ... who ... who understands."

Mitzi says, "You feel different."

Rafa laughs under her breath. "I am. I've let go of a lot of the little things, like my father's alcoholic absences, everyone disrespecting my mother, that prison of a school, and the know-it-all, do-nothing teachers and priests. And ... and ... this is Belatanu, my—um—boyfriend." Rafa is not sure how else to explain that they have talked about pledging to a year of consortship without having to explain much more besides. "He and Yuko-Hyun know all about you."

"Which means we all do," John says evenly.

"And this is my uncle Aaron Swanson, and my, um, step-grandfather John, and you know my mentor Doug, and this is Sarah, the, um, head of our Research Station, and Yuki's teacher Parvati; and Dora, Ella, and Selah, who, um, teach at the fertility school."

"We're all one big kindred in our community. Welcome to our kindred—and to Cascadia," Parvati says warmly.

"Would you like to try a waterslide?" Yukie asks.

"Yes!" Mitzi says.

Rafa and Mitzi give Doug a big hug before following Yukie in the direction of the slide and spa features, which are accessed through the education guild center in the southeast tower. Belatanu trails after them looking as if he is not quite sure of his ground. Yukie hangs back to speak with him, sending Rafa and Mitzi ahead to change into the soil-cleaned and shaken bark bloomers and tucked-in top they will use to enjoy the slide. After going down once, they climb up and do a series of dual slides in formations adapted from acrobalancing. The joy of movement, of reuniting with Mitzi, and of playing again as they did when they first met shifts the axis of Rafa's new world. She feels complete and infused with strengths new and old. Sarah and *Tío* are always talking about weaving the pattern of the future with the best warp threads of the past and the most promising they can invent and add; now she feels that she can reach back and gather all of the strands of light that have ever touched her with delight or love or serenity, and weave them into her life.

14

Nexus

W hen they have finished and rinsed off in the shower room, and are descending the spiral staircase toward their friends, Rafa stops, takes Mitzi's hand, and resolves to hold it as much as possible. "Look," she says, "there they all are, waiting for us. They all wish us here, and they all know how to deliver social joy as well as anyone can. We are both blessed to be here now."

"Don't you miss home?"

"This is home. I hope you'll feel that way soon. We could—we could do some kind of lifework together—with Belatanu—and with someone you choose."

"Crunch," Mitzi says warily.

"Too much too soon?"

"Uh—yeah!"

Rafa laughs, and the two friends rejoin the group and help prepare for a visit to the Customs House on the harbor, through which they can enter the outdoor market that is topped by a roof and enclosed by colorful hanging cloths. Rafa and Mitzi talk as they walk, holding hands. Mitzi talks of foraging her way west, of crossing the sand barrens at night and sleeping amongst the trees during the day. She stayed for a while at the Chaco Canyon historic site school campground, where she met a group of mushroom foragers and made friends with them. They agreed to teach her to find and disseminate several species. As they worked their way up the Green Watershed to the Snake, they were apprehended by the Mormon Genealogy Guardians and confined to a traveler's facility. Fortunately, Doug had put out a missing child notice for her, saying that she was sixteen, and the whole group was escorted to the trader's Guild Hall in Provo. She had been afraid at first, but they knew her full name and told her that her sister, Rafaela, was looking for her. Then she was hopeful enough to go with the next trader headed for Cascadia.

Rafa catches Mitzi up on all that has happened. She is pleased to find that Mitzi is fascinated by the vocations, and drawn toward the myth and reality of becoming a warrior. Rafa does not have to ask the reason; she too is troubled by pointless fears and nameless terrors. Becoming a warrior would mean coming to terms with risk, and with the limits of safety—especially in a community that understands safety as proactive, and as grounded in surviving, thriving habitats. Rafa promises to introduce her to Dirk.

When the young people have retrieved the crates of excess apples that they had brought on the boat, and Doug has arranged for Belatanu to sell them in the food section of the one-day part of the market, he leaves Bel with a laden cart and the women and invites the other men to the armory to watch a local hockey league game. As they walk away, Sarah calls out, "Wait!"

"For what?" Doug asks.

"Before you go, let's visit the Fairy Godmothers."

Doug looks baffled.

"We could have some fun with customers, and other people could enjoy them, too."

The dial in Doug's head comes to rest. He looks impressed. "What a good idea!"

"It happens," Sarah says wryly.

"Fairy Godmothers?" Rafa asks.

Yukie grins. "You'll see."

"What the hate?" Rafa laughs.

"No cursing, please," Belatanu says.

"Oh, right. What the love?"

Belatanu smiles, hands his cart off to Yukie, and cuts in between Rafa and Mitzi so that he is holding their hands. They go first to the one-day market, where he stays to sell apples amid the profusion of harvest stands that fill the yellow-curtained stalls of the food section. The others move on to the fuchsia-curtained stalls of the Fairy Godmother section, where Doug goes to a large counter behind which staffers are working at sewing machines with foot pedals, surrounded by racks that hold an astonishing variety of Hollywood-ized fairy costumes.

"I'd like a round of costumes, please, Jenny," he says, handing her his credit stick.

Jenny, a young woman in a pink, puffy-sleeved ballgown, hurries to the counter and eyes him sharply. "Is this a joke?"

"Nope."

She looks at Parvati and says skeptically, "Most of our customers are in the under-ten age group."

"We're young for the day," Parvati laughs.

Jenny shakes her head and smiles incredulously. "You must have made some big trades!"

"Always," Doug replies.

Mitzi and Rafa exchange a look of recognition. He is selling every way he can; the traders must be in trouble. Once Jenny has interviewed and measured each of them, and has taken estimates for Belatanu, she takes their wishes back to the seamstresses. Doug sends Sarah, her support team, Aaron, Parvati, and Yukie

to the Invention Section where they may find new instructional—
and sometimes practical—devices. Doug puts one arm around
Rafa and the other around Mitzi, saying, "I've been watching
you two. It looks like I now have two granddaughters with street
smarts. What do you say, Rafa, would Mitzi make a good trader?"

"I want to be a warrior!"

"Trading combines well with protection."

Rafa interjects, "We're both wondering why trading is down."

"Oh, that," Doug says with a grin. He adds more seriously, "I
think it's size. There's a right size for everything, and this market
is a little too small to serve the people who come to the Guild
Hall. The range of goods they want is so big, and the selection is
so limited, they go without or make their own or buy in Van. If
this were the only market center in the region—like Portland or
San Luis Obispo—the sellers and buyers would all come here."

"Maybe it isn't the right selection."

"Maybe. What do you think is missing?"

"I don't know. Let's look around."

Mitzi says, "Let's start with a treat."

"No food stands," Doug says. "Neighborhood politics. Too
many of the stores sell snacks and meals."

"There's one problem. They need to have stands and drum
up business."

"I agree. Tell the Fairy Godmothers when we go back for
our costumes. See if they can work some magic on the Guild
of Guilds."

They enter the daily part of the market, where Rafa and
Mitzi marvel at the beautifully crafted furniture, fun and imagi-
native sculptural wind generators, and handy baskets. They stop
at a kiosk that displays water baskets, where they notice that the
goods are unattended. Sales are all on the honor system, and are

overseen by one lone elder who is seated precariously on a stool, nodding as if about to fall asleep.

Mitzi says, "This market is backward. This is fancy store stuff. And if anyone came here, they'd lose half or more of it to theft. And nobody needs it every week."

Doug laughs to himself. "I should send you over to the market manager. He is stuck in his ways."

Rafa is listening with one ear while admiring the water baskets. There is one that looks like a pitcher that could go on her nightstand, where it would be practical and inspiring for its perfect handcrafting, elegant shape, and simple but striking high-contrast pattern. At the moment, she can't imagine living without it. All her lingering feelings of fear and insecurity clamor for the comfort of it.

"What does this mean?" she asks Doug as she examines the little green sticker on the pitcher's base.

Doug whistles softly. "That means it costs a hundred credits."

"A hundred!" she exclaims. "Who has that many?"

"Some of the elders."

"Do you? Would you buy it for me?" she wheedles, resting her head against his arm in comical pleading. "We've been through so much."

He grunts comically in return. "Oh, ho, ho. Don't try that with Belatanu. He'll lecture you about materialism."

"But you wouldn't."

"No. I'd lecture you about net gain vs. net loss."

Mitzi says, "You could see it as advertising. We could carry it around and talk it up."

"Nice try. Tell you what. I'll buy you a twenty credit gift as an incentive for going into trade."

Rafa looks at Mitzi. Mitzi raises one eyebrow; she looks

reluctant. Rafa says, "Let's see how much we can get and then split it."

"Yes."

"What?" Doug says, frowning.

"Looks like he doesn't know all about us!" Mitzi winks.

Doug laughs. "Guess not."

"Can we have some lines from your boat?" Rafa asks.

Half an hour later, Rafa and Mitzi have set up a ropes course on the buildings that line the pedestrian walk leading from the treasure-laden but drab daily market to the newly renamed Harbor Market Street. A crowd gathers before they finish and remains for their half-hour display of old routines. Rafa finds them unexpectedly easy. Perhaps it is the fertility guilders who have gathered with the rest of their group around the hat that Doug put out, and that is filling with market credit slips. Or, perhaps, it is the love between the friends that has always held them aloft. As they descend they notice a couple of Guild Guards standing by Doug, the broad brims of their Mountie hats covering their eyes, their hands on the hilts of their tranq guns. The crowd's applause, which the friends acknowledge with smiles and waves, dies away as they approach the hat, hand in hand.

The stern-looking Mountie says to his escort, "That's against the rules."

"Yeah. Too bad it's so hard to catch an acrobat."

"Yeah. Who can catch a gal who can leap tall buildings at a single bound?"

"I can't."

"I can't, either. We'll have to rely on this trusty elder of the trading guild to keep them in line. And to change those rules against having fun at the market." He winks at Doug, and they slip away.

"Keep your credits. I already bought it for you," Doug says in his best effort at a booming, triumphal voice.

Rafa looks a question at Mitzi, who nods happily. Rafa receives the basket from Doug with a wide smile, gives it to Mitzi with three air kisses, and then hands Doug the hat. "That's our contribution to the costumes. We lack for nothing now that you brought my missing sister-friend to be with us."

Doug's nose turns red; he is trying to hold back his emotions. Sarah hugs him tightly as the crowd applauds and whistles and then, group by group, peels away and flows once again to and from the market. When Doug has recovered his voice, he says gruffly, "Let's get the two of you and Belatanu back to the Fairy Godmothers before those mounties change their minds."

Half an hour later, after a raucous time in the changing rooms of Jenny's kiosk, Doug emerges as a pirate with a tall hat, eye patch, and pegleg; Sarah as a suffragette in bloomers; John as a zoot suit-wearing jazz man; Aaron as an old order Mennonite; Parvati as a professor in doctoral robes; Yukie as a voyageur in leathers; Mitzi as a trapeze artist in circus costume; and Rafa as a construction worker in a hard hat with dirt on her face. Ella, Selah, and Dora are clad as honorary Fairy Godmothers.

As they make their way back to the head of the harbor, explaining their costumes to curious passers-by and bubbling with laughter, Rafa asks Yukie what she found at the invention station. She takes something out of her pocket and puts her forefinger across her lips to signal silence, then bites her lips together to keep from laughing as she reveals a jointed bamboo snail. Mitzi looks at Rafa quizzically; Rafa shrugs. With a snap of the wrist, Yukie sends it flying forward toward Doug's hat. Another flick of her wrist, and the hat is in Yukie's hand. Doug puts his hand on his head and turns to look. With another flick, she puts it back on his head, where it sits askew.

"It's educational," she says by way of apology to the aston-ished Doug.

"The kids will love it!" Mitzi exclaims with a laugh.

"Are you sure that you want to give it to them?" Parvati asks.

"Not really," Yukie says, popping it back into her pocket.

As Belatanu catches up to them and it begins to drizzle, the young pull the old in the empty trader's handcart. After a wrong turn and a stop to ask a schooler for directions, they find the old stone cathedral where Doug wishes to eat lunch and exchange information.

The building is now a community spiritual center flanked by a multistory hot house kitchen garden dotted with single-person yurts. They leave the cart, enter the massive wooden doors at the front, and go through a foyer into the sanctuary. There they walk quietly so as not to disturb those who are praying or meditating in the pews and side chapels. Aaron admires the stark walls and high ceiling that set off the rose window of richly-tinted stained glass; the handsome carvings of the dark-stained, wood-wrapped chancel; and the colorful body of life embroidered on the altar cloth.

Doug leads them down the north aisle, from which Aaron admires the prayer benches and cushions of intimate side chapels. He notices that the ceiling of one chapel is covered by a celestial mosaic. The walls of another sport dazzling tapestries that depict Eden lands and wilderness restoration, and a third is hung with an array of bright blessing-covered ribbons that dangle from the ceiling to just above their heads.

He whispers to Rafa, "The churches in the Amanas are very

austere. This is … exuberant, effusive in comparison."

Rafa replies behind her hand, "It's like my mother's church, but hers is old style—stations of the cross, statues of bishops."

"I forgot that she was Catholic. Grandma grew up Lutheran —but gave it up for Judaism when we moved to the Amanas. She'd attend church on big holidays—like Christmas—to show respect. She didn't understand the Amana dialect, she just shared the spirit."

"Psst!"

Doug and John are waiting for them just beyond the altar. Aaron and Rafa and the others catch up as Doug leads them around the chancel to an old, peaked, wooden door wrapped in new iron-work. When Rafa opens it, warm air floods out and engulfs them in the sounds of voices and the arrhythmic clatter of metal plates and utensils. They descend the stairs and enter a hall filled with rows of long tables and benches where dozens of people in colorful jackets are eating and drinking and conversing.

Aaron asks, "Is this a … dining hall?"

"This is where they serve community meals—mainly for Betweeners."

"Who are they?"

"Travelers with no fixed home. They wear patchwork jackets to find each other—and to find temporary work."

"They're homeless?"

"Nomadic, I'd say. Most travel a circuit of churches until they settle somewhere for a while."

Aaron shivers at the remembrance of his years of self-imposed isolation in the comm tower, and the long, arduous, and perilous journey to this new life in which every day is a gift. "How awful!"

"The Betweeners I've met are like Léon," Rafa says. "They've lost their interbeing."

"I'd say they're passive: helpless and hapless, acted on and never acting," Doug says.

"They don't look well," John adds.

Doug says, "Most of the older ones worked old economy jobs. Sarah says they never learned to care for their energy bodies. They're wide open for exploitation and tend to give it all away."

"Like empties?" Rafa says.

"Empties can have strong energy," John says. "The Betweeners in Ithaca lack energy; they no longer fear the worst or hope for the best."

"They vary," Doug says.

They sit down and are soon waited on by Betweeners who are staying in the cathedral in a bunk room next to the dining room. The harvest menu includes squash sandwiches, corn, bean and yam salad, and other fall dishes unfamiliar to many of their group. When they have ordered and are waiting to eat, the Betweeners who are not eating rise like a flock of birds in patch-work plumage and come to light around their table to ask after the costumes, and then after those who are wearing them. Parvati compliments them on their curiosity. Aaron hears the fertility guilders gathering information on nearby barrens ready for the first stage of restoration; Sarah asking after stories of community renewal; John inquiring about local clinics; and Doug asking about everything and nothing.

When the food comes, those Betweeners go back to their places and others come to take their places. These are travelers-from a variety of communities; Aaron guesses that they are like a living comm network and decides to ask them about governance. He finds that while many communities they know have one leader or a group of elders from various guilds, others have taken their cues from the natural world, or from ancient history, or from the lessons of the intentional communities of the world. These are keen to know about the Amanas—so much so that he stops explaining his costume and starts telling the story of his prior home.

Soon, Sarah and her team leave for her nap on the boat, and all but Aaron and Doug leave to have tea at the greenhouse in the Park beyond the Provincial—now Cascadia—museum. Their heads are all buzzing with new information that they will each be able to discuss with others and perhaps use for the betterment of one project or another.

Left to themselves, Aaron and Doug walk north to the Armory to watch hockey. Doug asks, "Have you played hockey?"

"Never. Never even watched it."

Doug says, "I'll clue you in. And don't forget, information is a resource that's worth far more than apples or credits."

"That makes me a rich and generous man." Aaron laughs. "Thanks for the compliment."

Doug laughs. "You drive me as crazy as your mom did."

"You're welcome."

"Don't mention it. Please," he teases. "You're worse than John—he's only talking to her. You and Rafa are being her."

"John talks for her, too."

"Good point. You're all driving me nuts," he finishes with a smug grin that Aaron has, until now, only seen in pictures of Doug's college years.

When the sun has gone down, and all who sailed in on Doug's boat have gathered at the Empress Hotel for a meal in the games pub, John reunites with Gina and her wives, who have finished teaching their fertility classes and interviewing potential new wives. They are aiming for a group of five or seven, but object to something in each of their current candidates. They are not ready to risk what they have without feeling confident that things will turn out as they would wish. With them, John learns something every minute, and basks in their fertile care as they wait in the halls of the old hotel.

Even so, he has been dogged by wistfulness all day, which is leading him to tell Rafa and Mitzi his usual stories of the jazz and blues greats whom he heard, or met, or jammed with. He loves telling how they called him runner bean for his skinny body, and Gina loves pretending that he is telling it for the first time. He hopes that the young musicians from West Van with whom he will be playing tonight will not treat him like an antique or a museum, or idolize the lives and times of musicians, or hold other illusions that he cannot help but dash. If they do, they will divide him from the store of riffs that have come alive in his mind, and that will soon be still forever—unless Missy is right that they will survive the grave.

Doug, who is a welcome regular in this place, has arranged tables for them midway between the bocce court and snooker tables and the music stage. He has even arranged five extra seats, which John reads as a sign that guests or clients will be coming. When they have pushed their tables together, Doug says to Rafa, "See those curtains up there?" They all look up at the ceiling and the gauzy, colorful drapes that hang from it like an image of the aurora. "It's art and an incredible sound stopper. You can hear your friends talk. To enjoy the music without listening to games, you have to sit in the right place—which is right here."

John looks around at the crowd. Though sharply dressed, Gina and her wives look plain in comparison. Most of the guests are fantastically adorned in every kind of garb from sealskins to silks, and half stand out against the brightly-patterned easy chairs and sofas on which they sit as they drink and eat.

Rafa asks, "How do you know what your clients want for entertainment?"

"I find out and I provide it. Some want to strike a pose, some want to kick back, some want to cut loose. I can always figure out a way for them to enjoy this place."

Doug and Rafa take the group's orders and head to the food counter, wending their way around dartboards, table games, and floor games. They pause at the glass enclosure where culinary artists are carving butter and ice sculptures for the tables and creating castles of sweets for the dessert table. The counter staff soon fill platters with plates made of large leaves and cups and cutlery of pressed fiber. Servers will later follow with carts piled high with delicacies. As a classical guitarist goes to the stage to play, five strangers in vintage modern clothing come to the table and take the empty seats.

A middle-aged man with a waxed moustache who is wearing a suit from the 1890's says, "We know you, Rafa, and Aaron. We'll be coming to your fertility center for the enactments. I'm Gus, and this is Evelyn," he continues, indicating a round-faced young woman with big ears and a protruding chin, "and these are the Stein twins, Bob and Rob."

"We're not really twins," says Bob, who is short and round and half as tall as the towering, well-muscled Rob. "Rob and I came to hear John play. We've heard a lot of music—but never the hard-hitting blues and jazz from the period we specialize in."

"Come again?" John asks curiously.

"Each of us is an expert on a decade when the old economy went bust."

John wants to ask more questions, but Sarah cuts him off

and motions for Rafa to pull up a chair between her and John, opposite a sharp-nosed man of uncertain age with an elfin face marked by lines of sorrow. "Rafa, I want you to meet Caruthers. I asked him to look in on your father. I had no idea he'd be back from Denver so soon, or that he'd be able to pass on his news in person."

Caruthers holds up a pair of audio-visual spectacles and says in a thick brogue that John can barely decipher, "I filmed my talk with your da. You want to view it?"

Rafa hesitates and then takes the spectacles. She puts them on, and her limbs go loose, her expression vacant. After a few minutes, she looks disconcerted. Very gradually, she begins to cry. John can feel her heartache. "Are you all right?" he asks.

Rafa shakes her head and closes her eyes. "I ... I see the whole man. Usually I just see the part of him that causes me pain." Rafa removes the spectacles and hands them to Caruthers. "Thanks. That was ... unexpected. And welcome."

"Thank Sarah. I did it for her."

John asks, "How do you know her, and what do you owe her?"

"I'm with the Green School."

"Which is ... ?"

"Which is ... ?" Caruthers echoes dramatically. He raises his arms in a vee to draw the attention of all those seated nearby, and announces with theatrical incredulity, "We have a man here who's never heard of the Green School!"

"And one more," Rafa says.

Sarah laughs. "You've given Caruthers just the cue he was hoping for!"

Carruthers rubs his palms together. "You're in for a rare treat."

Doug interjects, "Can it, Caruthers. Give it to someone who gets to the point."

Evelyn says, "The Green School is our guild and traveling school. We live on the upper floors of the hotel and go out to communities who invite us to help them transition from the old economy to the new one."

Bob adds, "We go to the place and get to know it, involve the whole community in a theater camp, and then follow it with a silent retreat and a meeting for business. We help them create a new business incubator right on the spot."

Aaron says, "I'm surprised you stay here. This hotel can't be sustainable!"

"It can and is," says Gus. "There's a solar plant on the roof and a geothermal unit in the basement. What you see is the old shell."

"Like the Guildhall," says Aaron.

"And all the old buildings in town."

"What happens when the old panels fail?"

"Björn is going to take them. He'll remove the toxins and repurpose them."

"He doesn't know how to do that," Rafa points out.

"Yet," says Doug. "He'll figure it out. Or you or another initiate will."

"If he figures it out, the comm guild will want to know about it," Aaron says.

"He will, or someone else will. New methods are coming up like popcorn. And there's always Kilauea."

"It's more like a big game of leapfrog," Rob says. "We use that in our work with children. We show them that each community falls behind the rest until it leaps over the others, and they leap over it in turn."

"Nice image," Lena says.

"That's one way to teach them that timing is everything," Doug says.

"Why not send fertility teams with them?" Rafa asks.

"We do—if a community chooses restoration, or creative work."

"How many people have you reached so far?" Rafa asks.

"Counting towns that join our network, and people in those towns who do our practices—forty million or so, worldwide."

"How so many?" John asks.

"We encourage communities to help their neighbors."

"What are your practices?" Rafa asks.

The reply comes as a round robin. Gus begins by saying, "Our favorite is ground Reiki. When we—or another team—arrive in a place we find the main source of interbeing—"

Rob continues, "—which is usually a stand of trees or a group of people—"

Bob goes on, "and we replete the source."

Evelyn says, "We do that by gathering everyone who's willing in an old stone sanctuary or public building or natural amphitheater or dry quarry that isn't too magnetized."

Carruthers says, "And then we offer Reiki to the stone."

Gus finishes, "The stone stops all draws—and holds the energy of interbeing."

Rafa grins like Doug and says, "I'm beginning to see how you work."

"I don't see how you could energize stone," Aaron says skeptically.

"We don't need to know how it works," Sarah replies. "We only need to know that it does."

John muses, "It could be cosmic rays, gravitons, the ionosphere, sunspots—"

"Or the illusion of control," Doug grins smartly. "We rationalize things to convince ourselves that we matter when we don't."

Sarah says to Rafa, "We learn from life by noting any discord between the ideal and real, and by resolving it in favor of the real."

"Mom used to say that life leads," Aaron says, "and that concepts follow."

Yuko-Hyun, who has been squirming with impatience, interjects, "When will you play? I want to hear the music Sarah's been telling us about."

John lifts his eyebrows, then gets up and bows with impish formality, motioning for Gina to stay where she is. He walks over to the green room and introduces himself to the musicians. They barely notice him at first; they are too busy arguing the fine points of baroque ornaments and disputing the best source of virtual instruments. After a time, John joins in the conversation. His heart lifts. He is with musicians, and he finds himself coming to life. After a time, they turn the conversation to jazz and blues artists, and debrief him as they would any new stand-in. Soon he is going on and on about his adventures in Chicago and points east. When he tells of seeing Baden Powell at the Blue Note, the guitarist goes green with envy.

Their conversation circles the globe, and John learns more about music than he has done in decades. By the time they have run through the program and set a few chord progressions and solo rotations, he is flying high, and so is the group. They file onto the stage, and the front man announces a program of traditional classics. They play Aaron Copland, Cole Porter, Duke Ellington, John Coltrane, Muddy Waters, and Chick Corea, and then improvise like Ornette Colemans' group—each playing what he or she pleases at once. The audience is rapt; they give all of their attention to the players, and the players turn it into a dialogue. John suddenly realizes that this is how Gina and her wives want to make love.

Acknowledgments

I am grateful for this book—and for my life—to the individuals, groups, and movements that have revealed that the anthropocene age is poised to end life on Earth. With respect to poisoning, I thank: those providers who have stepped up to help patients as best they can when medicine as a whole failed the chronically poisoned; Rachel Carson and all who heeded her book *Silent Spring*; and the activists who agitated for shielding of microwave ovens. With respect to human dispersal of organisms that unbalance habitats, I thank Elizabeth Kolbert and the scientists whose work she has disseminated in her book *The Sixth Extinction*. With respect to consumptive destruction of the body of life that creates the biosphere that gives life to all species, I thank the indigenous people who set our species a good example, and the theologians and philosophers who teach unitive thinking.

I am indebted to the sentinels of the emerging paradigm that laid the groundwork for doctors of life, and to specialists in preventive medicine and public health for keeping alive the contextual and complex thinking introduced to medicine by Hippocrates and reduced to statistical modeling in my time as an academic, and David Sackett and others who formalized the "N of 1" studies of and by individuals in partnership with their doctors.

With respect to our species' history of extinction, I thank Michael Wood and the BBC for their coverage of the loss of the Indus Valley and Eridu civilizations to the consequences of urbanization on the environment, as well as to archaeologists who have noted that deforestation in the British Isles began almost with the end of the last ice age and the North American extinction—by humans—of the mastodon.

I am also grateful to the many artists and thinkers who have brought the problem to attention, especially Columbus, James Fenimore Cooper, Thoreau, Lawrence, Tolkien, David Suzuki, Lin Onus, Wendell Berry, Charles Mann, the scientists who document extinctions, and—with respect to the shadow side of medicine—Mary Shelley and Robert Louis Stevenson.

Last and not least, I am grateful to the Southern Oregon team that made this book beautiful. The appearance is due to the professional competence and creativity of cover artist Bruce Bayard and book designer Chris Molé. The readability is due mainly to coach Chansonette Buck and editors Deidre Krupp, Deborah Mokma, and Ann DiSalvo.

Such writing ability as I am developing, I owe first to my father, who taught me reading and writing at a young age. I am also grateful to editor friends Eva Silverfine and Stephanie Holt for their talent and skill in verbal expression, and to writing teachers Andrea Goldsmith of the Victorian Writer's Centre and Wendy Call of Hugo House. They kindly put up with an unusual and neurotoxic student, trusting that their wisdom would not go to waste.

Thank you also to my book development and beta readers, especially: Jan Agosti, Anna Barón, Jessica Bondy, Cynthia Bradley, Julie Clayton, Stephanie Holt, Christopher Howell, Joel Mason, Sara Myers Wade, Berta Nicol-Blades, and Dana Smaller. Special thanks to Jan, Ann, Julie, and Stephanie for their kindness in dark times.

About the Author

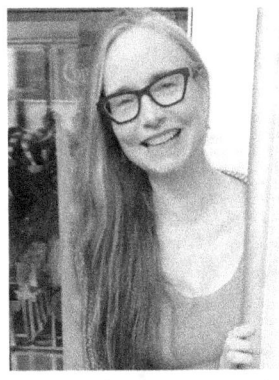 **Beth Alderman,** MD, MPH earned her AB and MD degrees from the University of Chicago and her MPH from the University of Washington. After Board Certification in Preventive Medicine and Public Health, she took a faculty position in the University of Colorado Medical School Department of Preventive Medicine, Biometrics, and Medical Informatics, where she did population-based epidemiological studies of adverse reproductive outcomes and methodological studies in clinical epidemiology. In her next faculty position at the University of Washington School of Public Health, she focused on risk factors for birth defects.

In 1996, she fell ill with the mysterious new plague and was given the provisional diagnosis "chronic fatigue syndrome". She has spent her time since studying her own case and pondering the reasons that her beloved profession failed her so completely. Fortunately, she discovered her cure, which may be of use to others suffering from one or more of the emerging epidemics affecting humans, their habitats, and life on earth.

For more about and from the author, see the following websites:

BethAldermanMD.com	*Free Information for all readers*
DoctorsOfLife.com	*For care and cure of all lives as one*
LivingFutureBooks.com	*Publishing Website*
LivingFutureCourses.com	*Educational Website with Free and advanced Courses*

Look for author's books on Amazon.com

Other Books by
Beth Alderman

Medical Phenomenology:
Chronic Ambient Poisoning

ISBN: 978-1-7332849-2-9

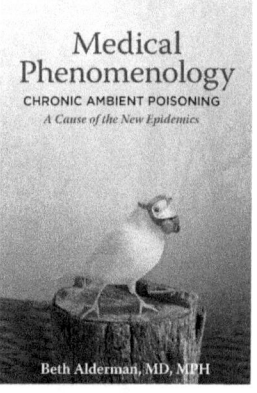

One day in December of 1996, the author (a physician, medical detective, and academic epidemiologist) developed disabling brain fog following on a decade-long descent into a painful, pervasive, and unprecedented chronic illness. Having done population-based studies to research the causes of birth defects, and having thus encountered the limitations of modern methods, she had inadvertently prepared to investigate the causes of her illness—which was given the provisional and uninformative label of "chronic fatigue."

The author began a delineation of the natural history of her condition using the methods of: doctors Hippocrates, Maimonides and Oliver Sacks; the "radical empiricism" used by Dr. William James; and the phenomenology introduced by Teilhard de Chardin and Merleau-Ponty. After a fifteen-year search, she found a doctor of integrative medicine whose elimination diet relieved her brain fog, which enabled her to complete a self-study and to construct an actionable new diagnosis: chronic ambient poisoning. Unseen by doctors and obscured by medical dogma and a myriad of false diagnoses, chronic ambient poisoning defies late modern, fragmented, accuracy-challenged medical research methods and delivery systems. It also reveals that human-caused habitat injuries that afflict birds, bees, and other species are affecting humans while driving evolved life toward extinction in the way of an asteroid strike. To ignore this diagnosis is to ignore the dangers to all lives posed by maladaptive modern lifeways.

The Evolve Fertility Series

BOOK 1
Melissa's Match: *Great Society*
ISBN: 978-1-7321110-1-1

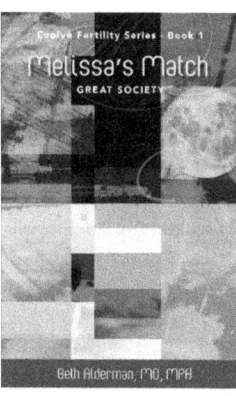

It's the early 1970s. Melissa and her friends begin their first year of college in the inner city of Chicago at a time when post-assassination riots, Great Society scholarship programs, and veterans returning from Vietnam create a sometimes explosive confluence of urban and rural, rich and poor, white and black, educated and uneducated. Coming of age in a violent, unjust, and yet hopeful time, they struggle to reconcile their hopes and opportunities with the shadows of war and the destructive clashes of senescing and emerging systems of care and cure of life on earth.

BOOK 2
Connie's Conception: *Awareness of Peril*
ISBN: 978-1-7321110-0-4

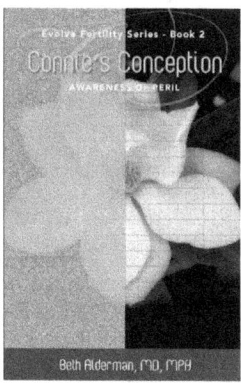

It's the late 1980s, and Connie Martin, a doctor working for the Epidemiology Intelligence Service of the CDC, is called to Colorado to investigate an alarming outbreak of birth defects. Born illegitimate in the San Luis Valley as Consuela Martín, a name known only to close friends and to her beloved gamer and programmer husband, she arrives as an unknown. Joined by environmental activists who suspect the state's Superfund sites and by doctors and parents who fear for its children, Connie attempts to discover the link between habitat destruction and damage to innocents.

BOOK 3
Melissa's Malady: *End of Modernity*
ISBN: 978-1-7321110-2-8

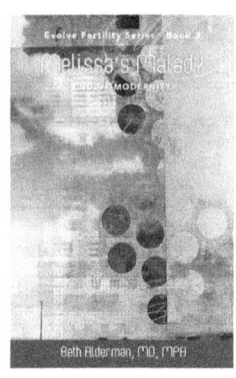

IIt is almost the year of the millennium, and Melissa meets her college friends Sarah and Doug and her first and only true love John for a reunion in Hyde Park. All four are in the midst of their careers. All struggle with the compromises that have marred their happiness. All wish to change the world, each in a different way. Sarah has left her government job for a new life as a yoga teacher. Doug is helping to birth a new value-based economy. John is a successful academic doctor. Melissa is ailing. They unite to turn John's success as a researcher to the cure of Melissa's mysterious chronic illness. What they find will change their lives and their imperiled world.

BOOK 4
Colette's Creativity: *Sacred and Profane*
ISBN: 978-1-7321110-3-5

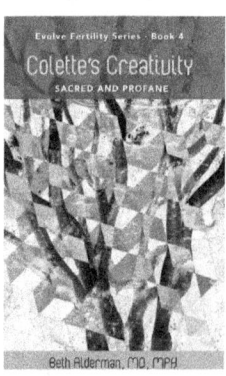

Colette, Melissa's childhood friend, abandons her marriage and home in Maine and flies to Melbourne. There she is taken in by her friend Reggie, who seems to know the secret of joy. Colette joins in the lives of striking individuals who lead her to view sexuality as a manifestation of the sacred. As she leaves behind the wounds caused by profane sexuality, she and her new friends clash with members of Reggie's family who force them to flee and to begin again.

BOOK 5
Colette's Community: *Thirds*
ISBN: 978-1-7321110-4-2

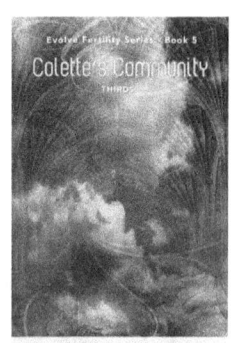

Soon after Colette and her friends find a new home, an old boyfriend of Melissa's who is sojourning in Australia calls and expresses his desire to visit. Colette plans to use the visit as a chance to develop a job for herself; he plans to check up on Colette for Melissa. As they get to know each other, they see that despite differences in religion, origin, and experience, they are on very similar spiritual paths. When it is time for Randall to go home, Colette joins him in Chicago. When he becomes caught up in his old life, however, she returns to Australia to pursue her dream of giving birth to a sacred community.

Chronic Illness Owner's Manuals
Regenerate Your Life: Chronic Illness as a Springboard for Creating Your Best Life

ISBN: 978-1-7321110-8-0 (VOL. 1)

ISBN: 978-1-7321110-9-7 (VOL. 2)

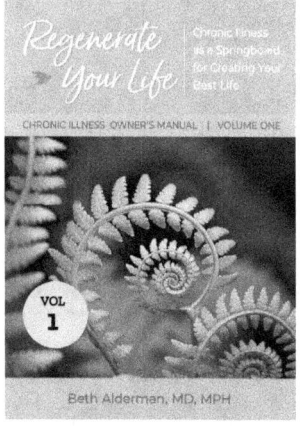

The *Chronic Illness Owner's Manual* series is for patients with chronic illness, and for the people who care for them. Suitable for individual or small group use, it offers a comprehensive, systematic, step-by-step approach to engaging modern medical systems, and to healing from the inside out.

The books comprise anecdotes, exercises, and quotes that address recovery through seven aspects of the body: awareness, understanding, perceptions, sensations, energy, flesh, and interbeing. The frames, constructs, patterns, and processes employed by the series are drawn from traditions of medicine, field biology, theology, and psychology from around the globe. Their synthesis offers an emerging, sustainable, eco-centric, eco-contextual, and customizable approach to creating a new and better life that regenerates your unique meaning, purpose, and vision of abundant life. The *Chronic Illness Owner's Manual* series complements care and cure courses available online at www.LivingFutureCourses.com.

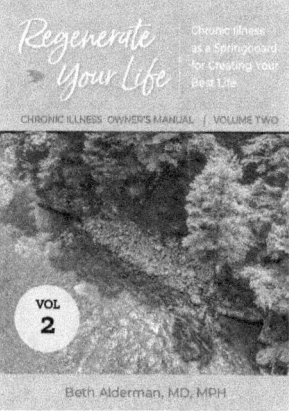

The Evolve Restoration Series
Sequel to the Evolve Fertility Series

BOOK 1
Pilgrim Minds: *After the War on Life*
ISBN: 978-1-7321110-5-9

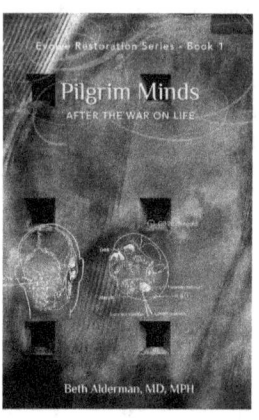

Melissa's deathbed request catapults her son Aaron on a journey from her family's Mississippian clinic to the Salish Sea to claim a mysterious legacy. Meeting his niece Rafa en route, he continues overland with her, and uncle and niece come to know and depend on each other. On arriving at the Saltspring Island Research Center (SIRC), Sarah, now the keeper of the center's narratives, confesses that Aaron's legacy is a task: to apply his mother's philosophy to SIRC's lifeways in order to revitalize it.

While he had been immersed in his mother's medical philosophy, SIRC had used many of her ideas to found a fertility school. SIRC's encroaching apathy persuaded Sarah that they missed one or more essential lifeways, and hopes that Aaron may be able to pinpoint and provide them. Taken by surprise, but ready to step up, Aaron immerses himself in the community, and Rafa undergoes SIRC's initiation process. Uncle and niece come to love Cascadia and to relish local, burgeoning patterns of innovation. Both choose to stay at SIRC, an agentic community that is doing much to restore evolution and its living future.

BOOK 2
Aaron's Legacy: *The Body of Life*
ISBN: 978-1-7321110-6-6

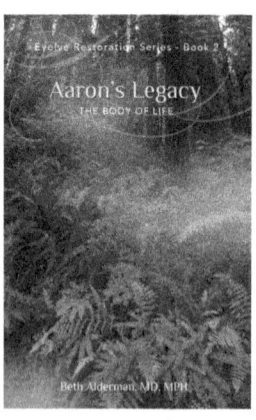

Having come to know the community, Aaron receives his legacy as a series of enactments of SIRC's history. The surviving members of his mother's old friendship group—Sarah, Doug, and John—join the audience and performers in processing and adapting their shared narrative. In the intervals between enactments, Rafa undergoes initiation while Aaron explores the composer, an instrument that enables a player to evoke memories with images and to express the player's responses as sound scapes. As Aaron shares his with Rafa, Sarah and others, John shares memories of Melissa, and seems to receive a new message from her.

As the community adapts to changes in its meaning and purpose, Rafa and Aaron each finds a first consort and draws inspiration from local knowledge keepers and change agents residing at SIRC, the nearby Monastery of Origins and Endings, or in Victoria or Vancouver. Aaron's health, damaged by his travel through a poison barren, deteriorates. With his death, his consort Parvati shares their legacy in the form of patterns of action that may remove roadblocks to continuous adaptation and renewal.

BOOK 3

The Kindred's Rebirth: *Rough Seas and Far Lands*

ISBN: 978-1-7332849-3-6

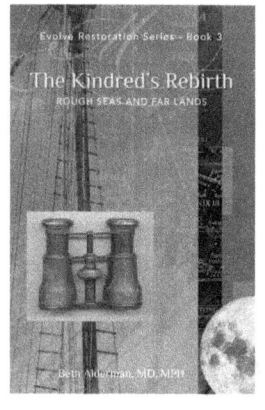

A decade later in Australia, Parvati and Björn give up on effecting meaningful restoration there. Dirk, while on his annual circuit of the north, arrives in Jokkmokk for the annual Sámi gathering to learn that SIRC is in crisis. Rafa, who is crossing the South Pacific on her two year global clinic circuit, hears strange news: the Fertility School, which was winding down, closed without notice. She realizes that her work, too, is drawing to a close as her clinics adapt to localism and begin to diverge.

All three travelers feel a strong homing urge and hatch a plan to converge in Scandinavia with the remnant of the SIRC community. En route, Parvati adopts a grandchild, Jacki, who helps Björn to recover from a disorder of interbeing. Many new consort pairs join the kindred and revive it by helping to form a next community, SIRC-Umea, and to organize and maintain residential restoration communities in the Baltic and North Sea bioregions, and to recover from the painful loss of the original community.

BOOK 4
Jacki's Vision: *The Green Line*
ISBN: 978-1-7332849-4-3

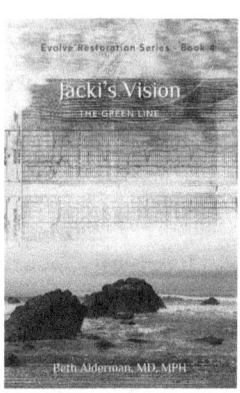

When Jacki turns sixteen, she begins her transition to adulthood by venturing into larger worlds of knowledge and adaptation to gain skills. During her first clinic circuit in the Baltic, she finds that her coming of age is coinciding with her kindred's restiveness. As she embraces and contemplates her future, a vision takes hold of her. She proposes a Green Line restoration project in Tasmania to reconcile a time debt created by the Black Line genocide, and to prepare her for organizing bioregional restoration projects. Her kindred and their networks embrace the project, expand it, and multiply its potential effects.

As the Green Line Corps prepares to depart en masse for Tasmania, Jacki meets a young stranger, Mirek, whose experience of the world—whose very umwelt—contrasts with her own. Later, in Tasmania, she gains a consort, Izaak, and a sister friend, Lally, both of whom winnow her possible futures. Together, the many thousands of Green Line participants develop a restoration ethos and synchronize living processes for restoring habitats—with their restorers. Jacki and her new peers are among the first to return to the original SIRC campus, near which many former kindred members have settled, and to which many others are about to return.

BOOK 5
Mel's Motherhood: *A Place in the Living World*
ISBN: 978-1-7332849-5-0

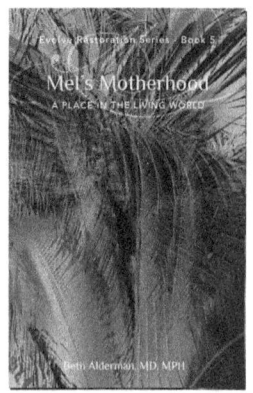

Mel and JJ—children of the Three Mammas—await the advance boat from Tasmania at the Cascadian Monastery of Origins and Endings. Mel, who is pregnant, and JJ, who fared poorly while he was away, finished their initiation projects and are keen to see Jacki and to meet the new kindred members. In the course of a joyful reunion, Mel and JJ learn that Jacki and Lally are also pregnant.

As this next generation of adults chooses ways to express fertility and defines new vocations, the reconstituting kindred celebrates new human lives, integrates with local communities, and processes hitherto hidden threads of SIRC's history with the aid of DNA fathers who participate. The complex, complementary communities adapt to continuous learning via phenomenology, and to continuous adaptation of systems for care and cure of evolved life.

Meaningful Retirement: *Become a Life Care Provider*

ISBN: 978-1-7332849-0-5

Meaningful Retirement is a self-guided monthly course in four seasons that can aid people like you who are exiting modern employment or withdrawing from the modern death economy. In it you will find a toolbox for transition to a vocation of life care, and thus begin to mature into a wise elder able to lead and mentor those who follow you. These seasons include:

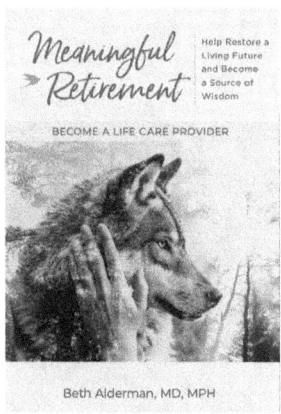

- **A Summer Breather**
- **A Fall for Reflection**
- **A Winter to Reclaim Your Personal Narrative**
- **A Spring for Revolutionizing Your Lifetime Learning**

As you transition to the role of provider of life care, you may choose to co-found emotionally and spiritually astute communities where you can mentor your juniors, who face the imminent and daunting task of passing through wrenching psycho-social change while arresting and reversing the accelerating human-caused Sixth Extinction. That threat to evolved life represents a unique crucible for transforming modern lifeways into ones that enable humans to choose and to restore life. Re-visioning and co-creating processes of care and cure that restore all lives as one will prepare your species to restore the planet's living lungs, its water circulation, its living shade, and its evolved resilience to unexpected planetary catastrophes. By viewing life in time though an eco-centric and eco-contextualized lens that scales from your lifetime to evolutionary time, you can begin to see your world through new eyes that reveal your place in the big picture of life on earth.

Direct learning, that is, phenomenology, is essential for restoration of a living future. This method has changed with every epoch since ancient natural historians began to attempt to create views, frames, and constructs in an attempt to grasp evolving generative systems. The present moment of peril can be taken as an impetus and inspiration to engage with an exciting process of learning and problem solving that some call the living paradigm. This paradigm, which is still incubating in fields as diverse as architecture and design, agriculture, archaeology, restoration, and theology, is ripe for grass roots syncreses across outdated fields of knowledge. When you learn to cooperate with the last hundreds of millions of years of evolution while pursuing space age ways of averting asteroid collision, you will be prepared to lead your species toward sustainability and to make room for rapid human adaptation that restores evolution. Welcome to the One Life..

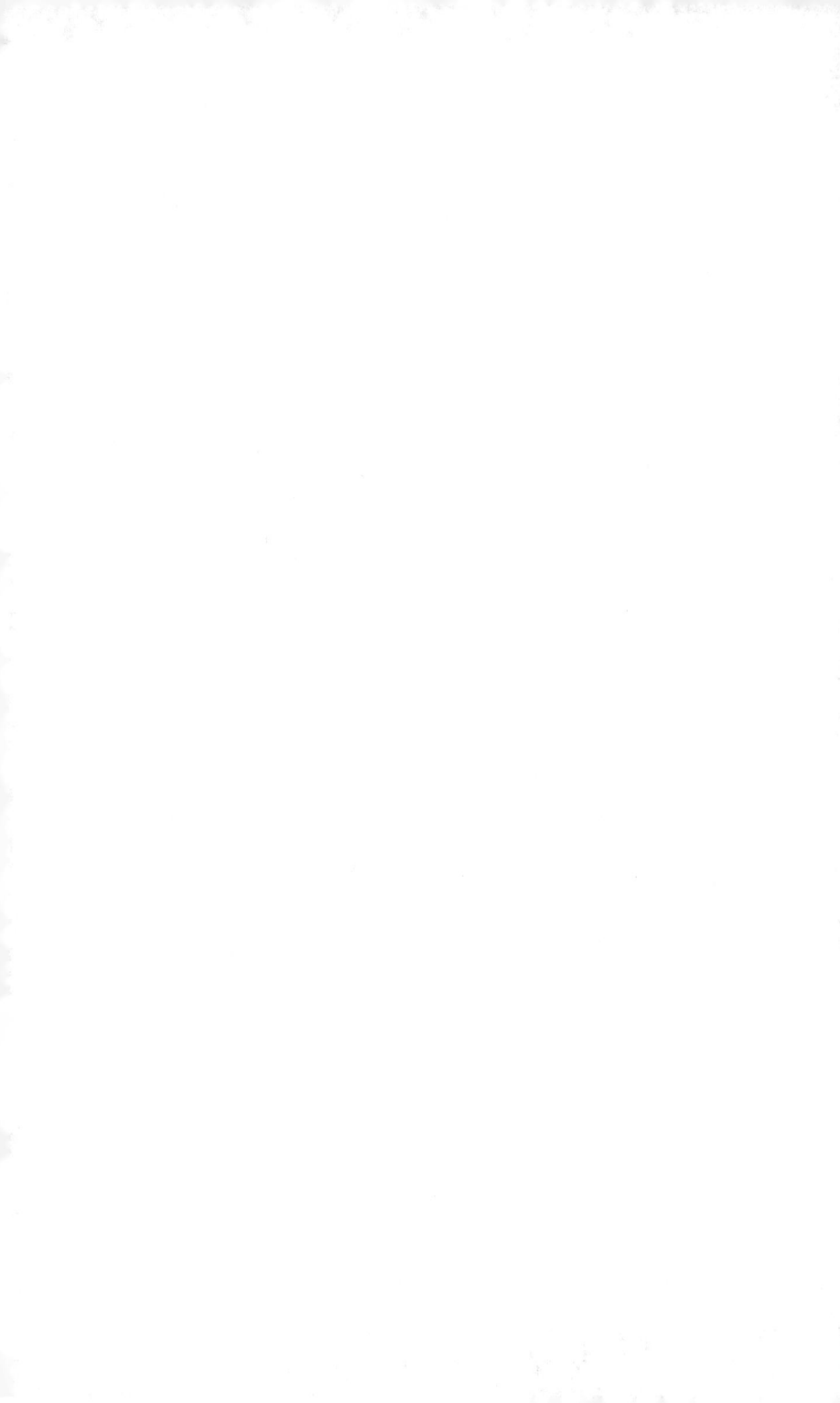